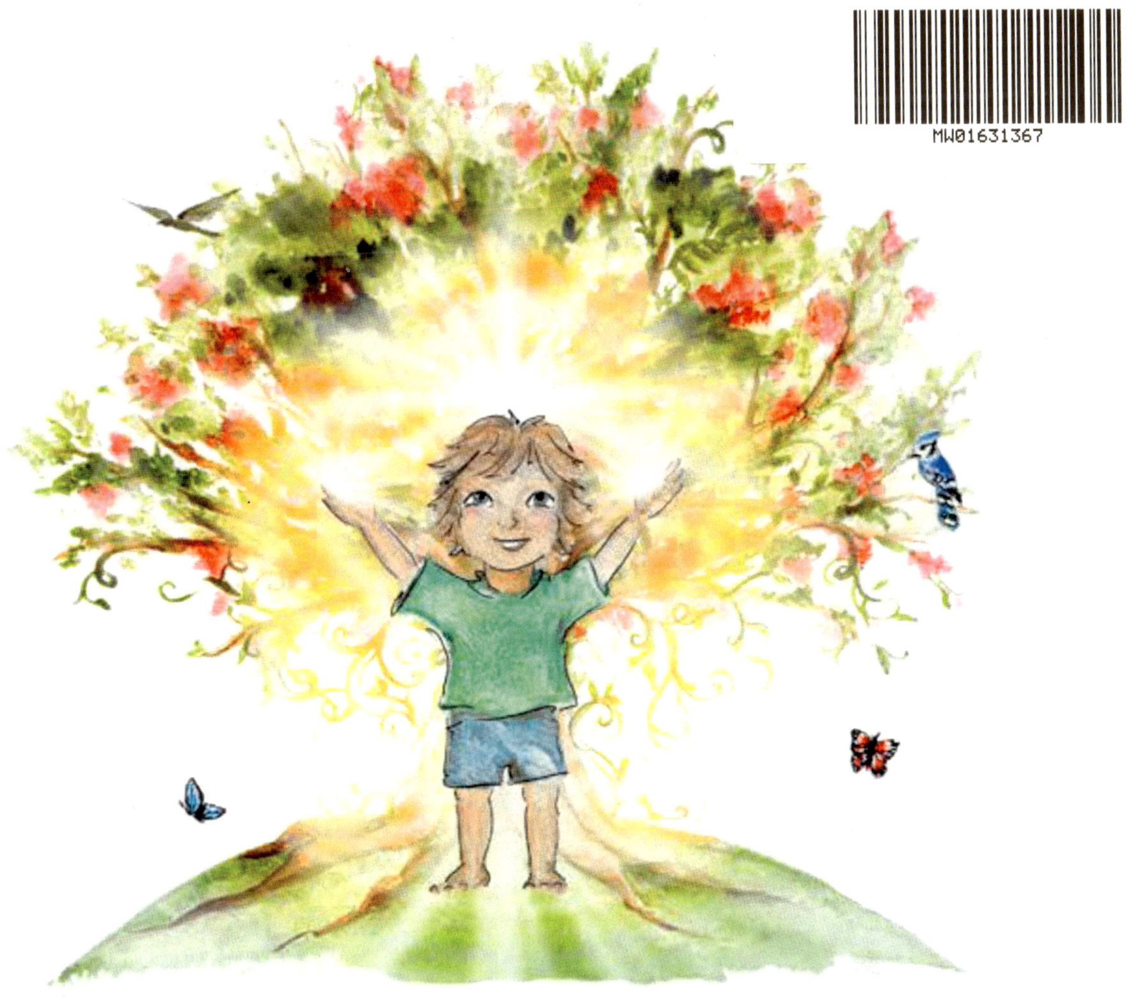

Printed in the U.S.A.
Published by Two Penny Publishing
850 E Lime Street #266 Tarpon Springs, FL 34688
TwoPennyPublishing.com | info@twopennypublishing.com

For permission requests and ordering information, email the publisher at: info@twopennypublishing.com

ISBN: 978-1-950995-99-8

FIRST EDITION

For more information about the author or to book event speaking
or appearances, event or media interview, please contact:
info@twopennypublishing.com

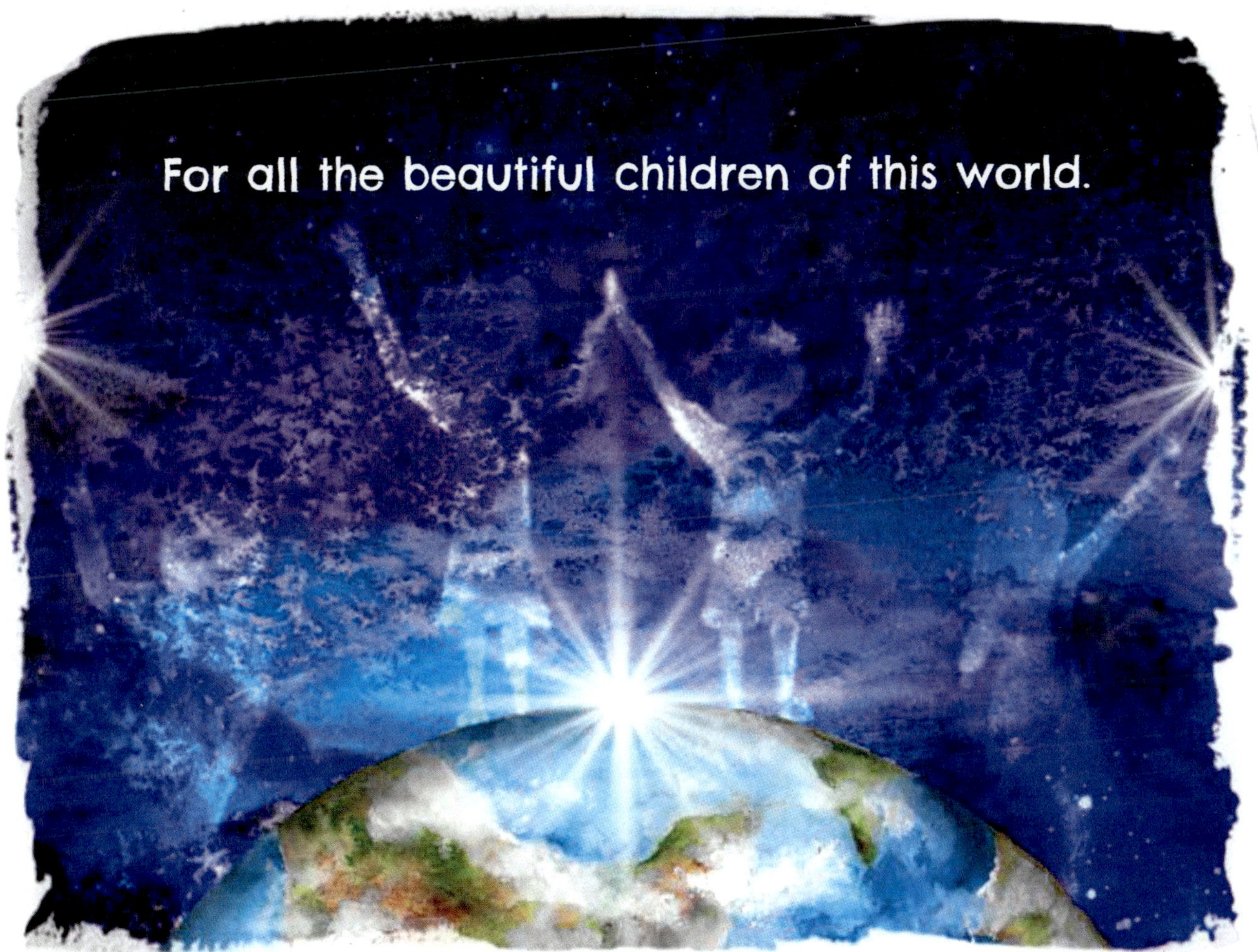
For all the beautiful children of this world.

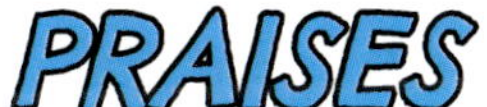

PRAISES

This is a simple but beautifully written book about how incredibly smart the human body is. Children will learn that their body is naturally capable of health & healing, and this provides a simple to understand explanation to start them on their journey.

Dr. Pamela Stone McCoy ICPA Instructor

Dr. Patty wrote a brilliant book for children to learn and remember how extraordinary the innate wisdom is within the body.

Anne Ribley, author and host of the Remarkable Souls Podcast

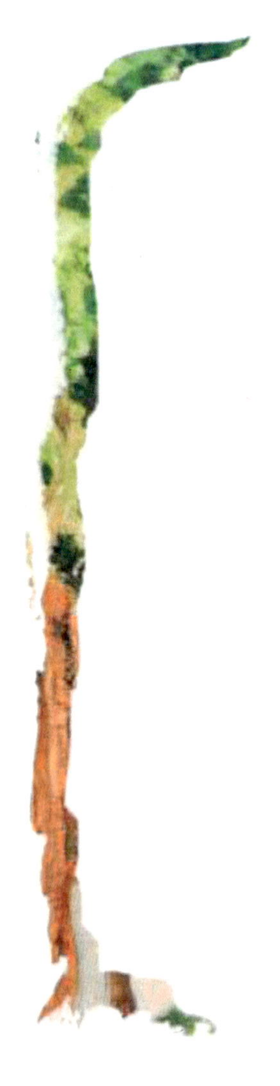

My body is the most

AMAZING

thing because of

how smart it really is.

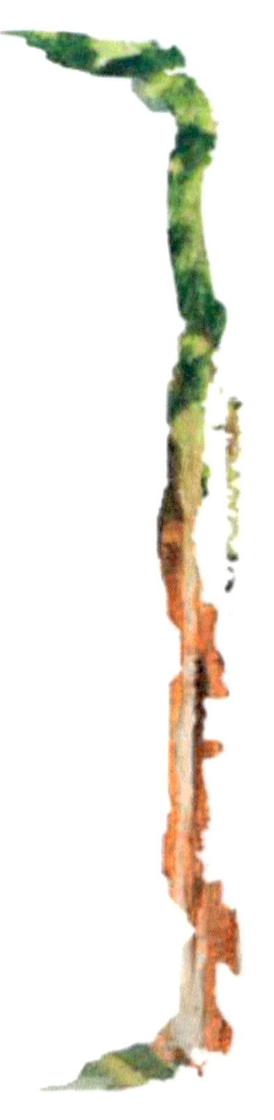

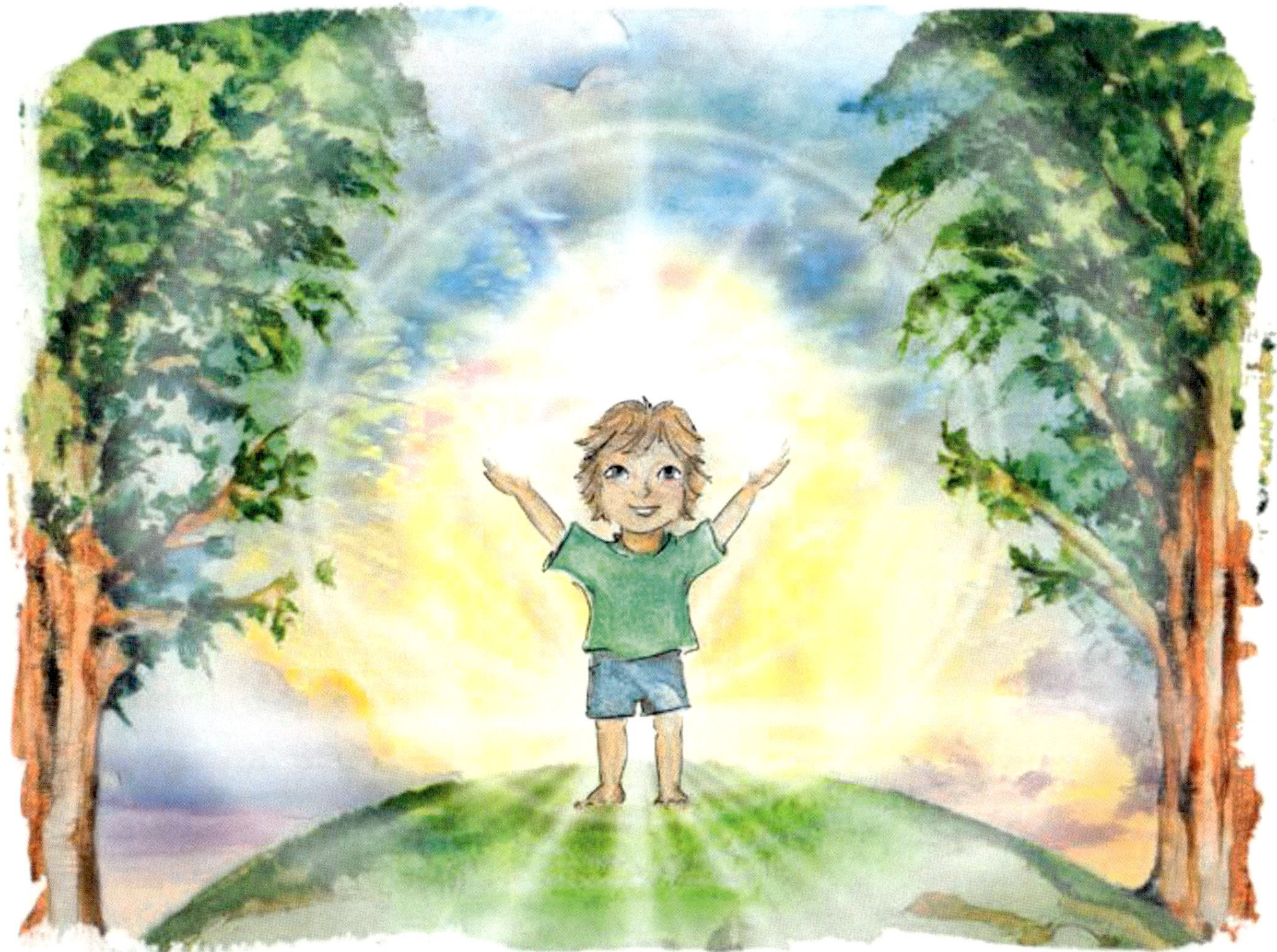

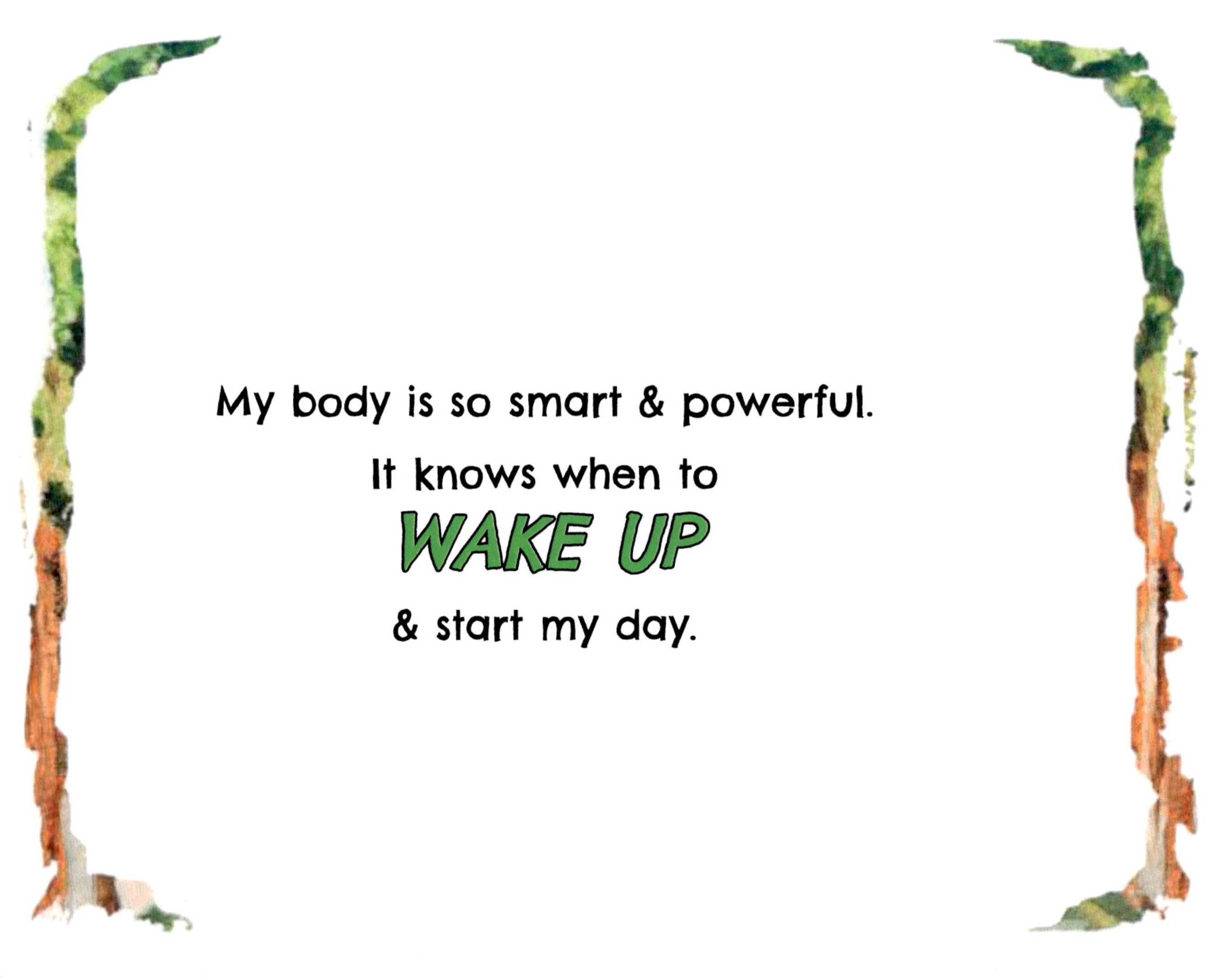

My body is so smart & powerful.

It knows when to

WAKE UP

& start my day.

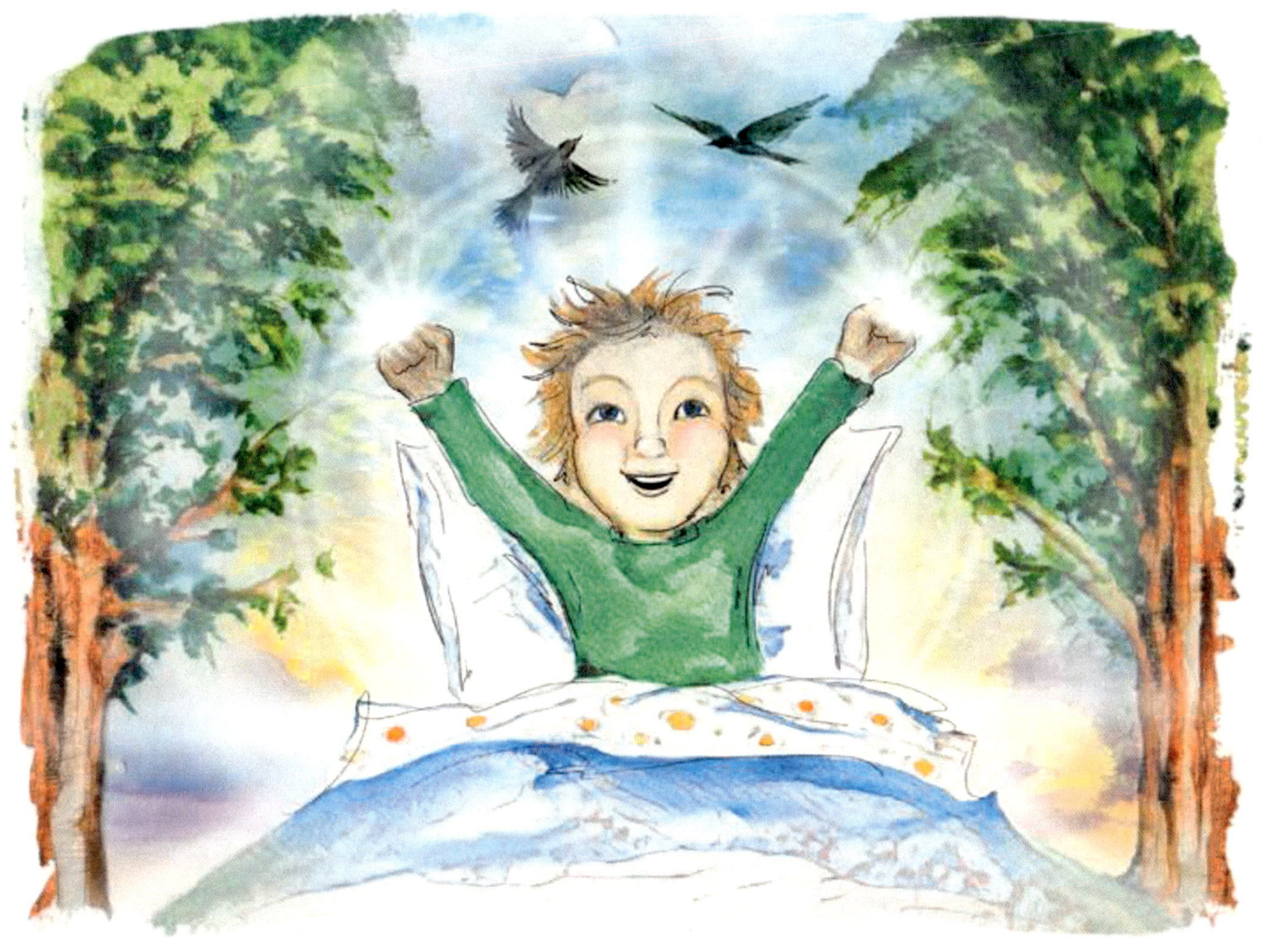

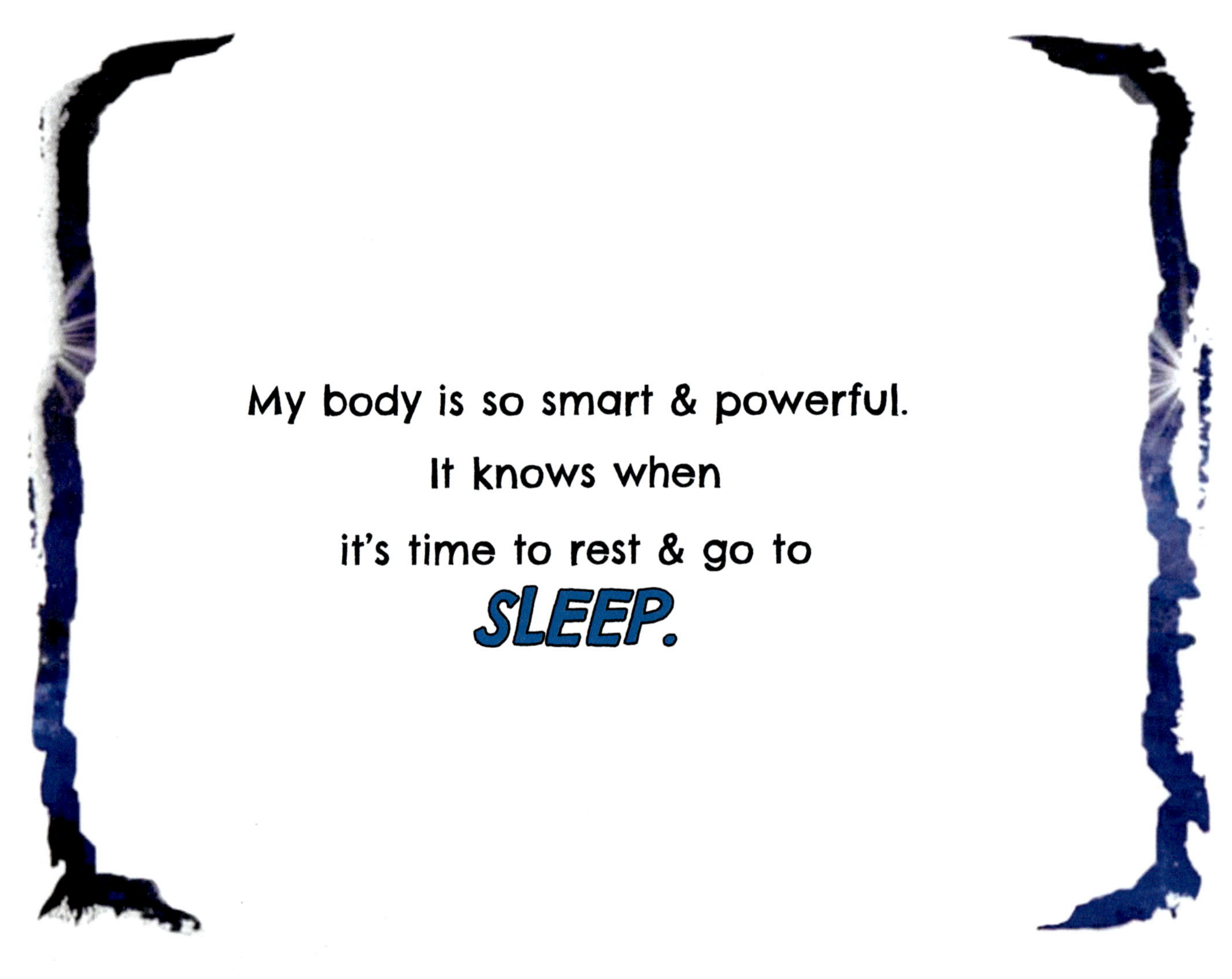

My body is so smart & powerful.

It knows when

it's time to rest & go to

SLEEP.

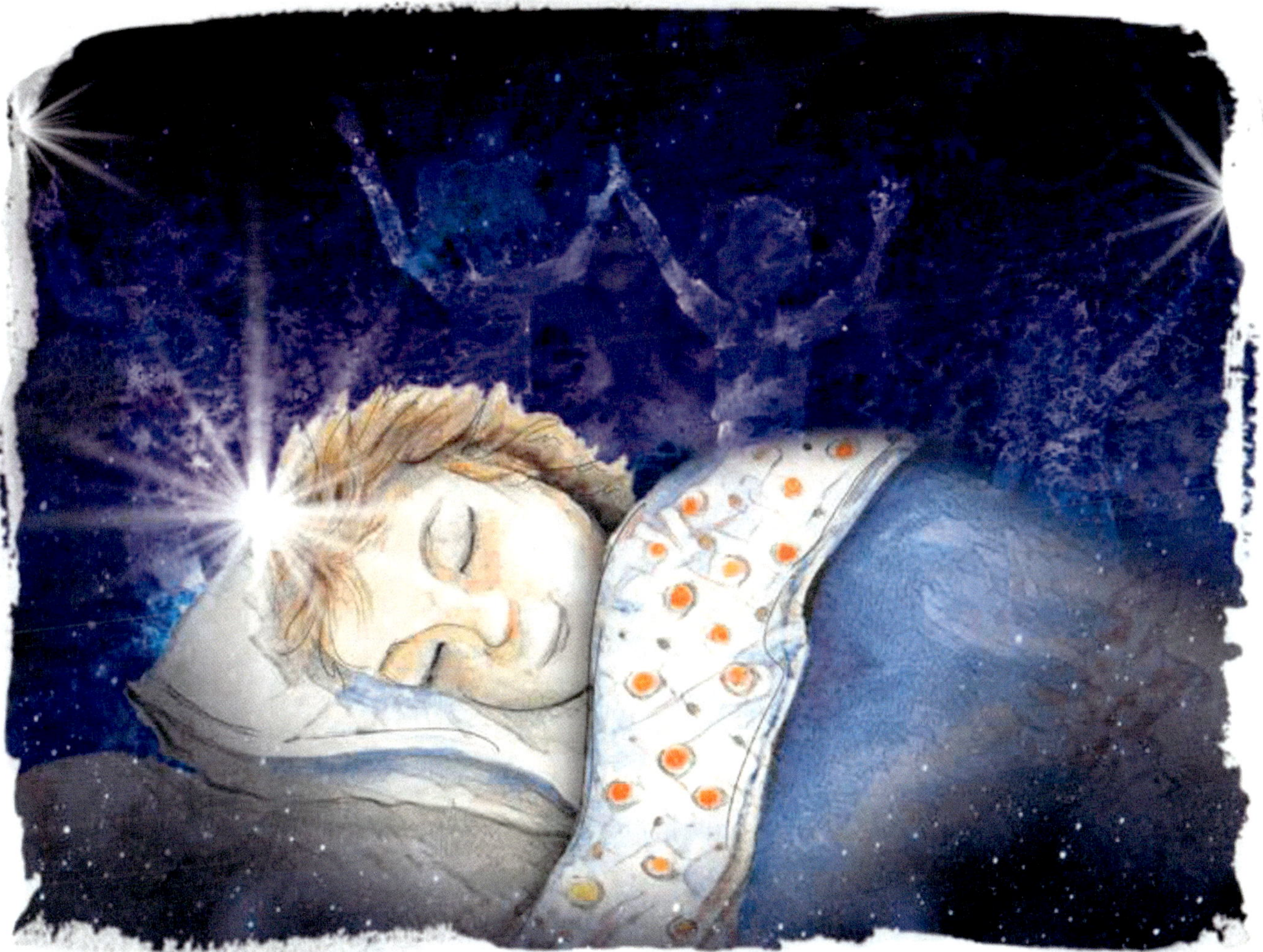

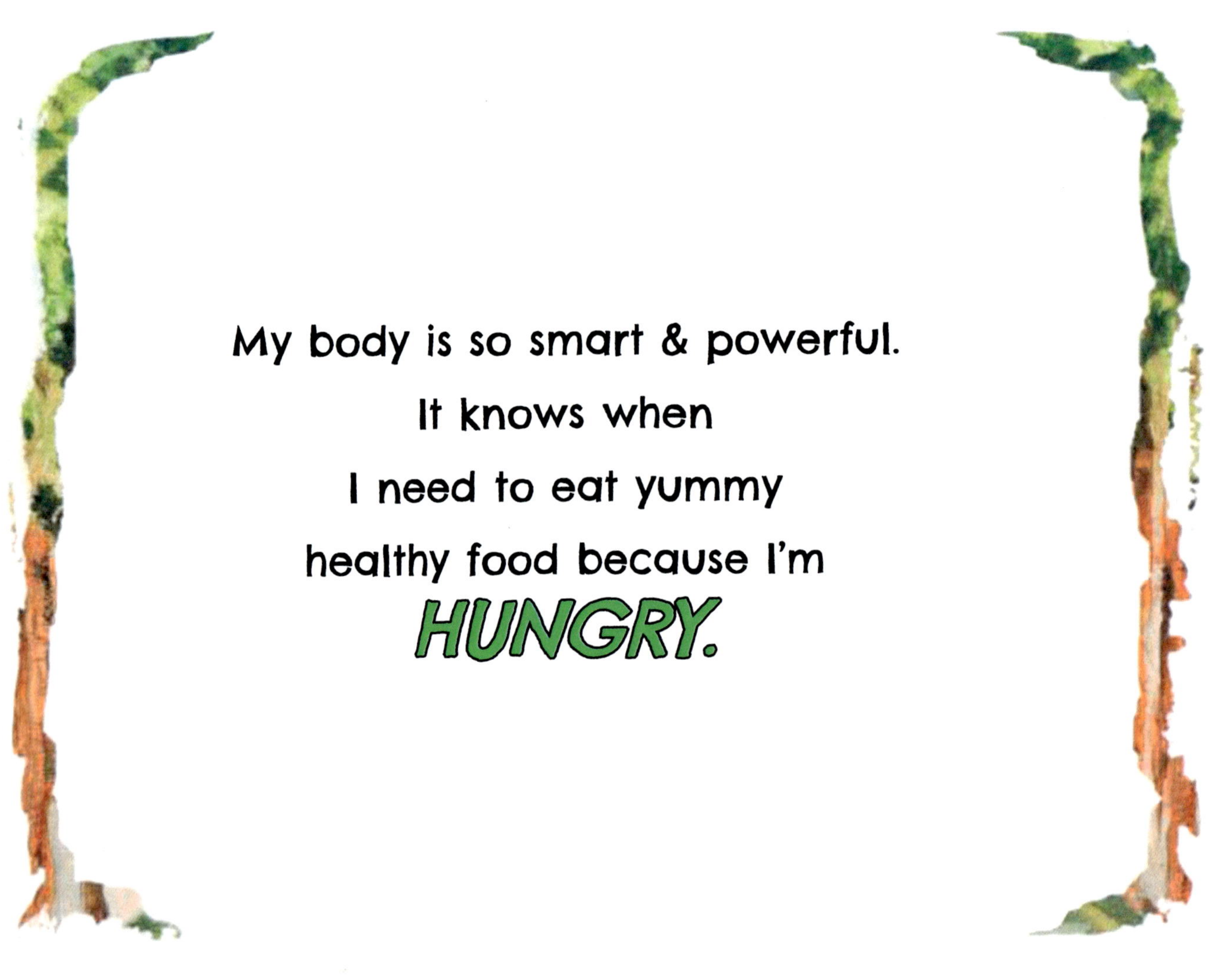

My body is so smart & powerful.

It knows when

I need to eat yummy

healthy food because I'm

HUNGRY.

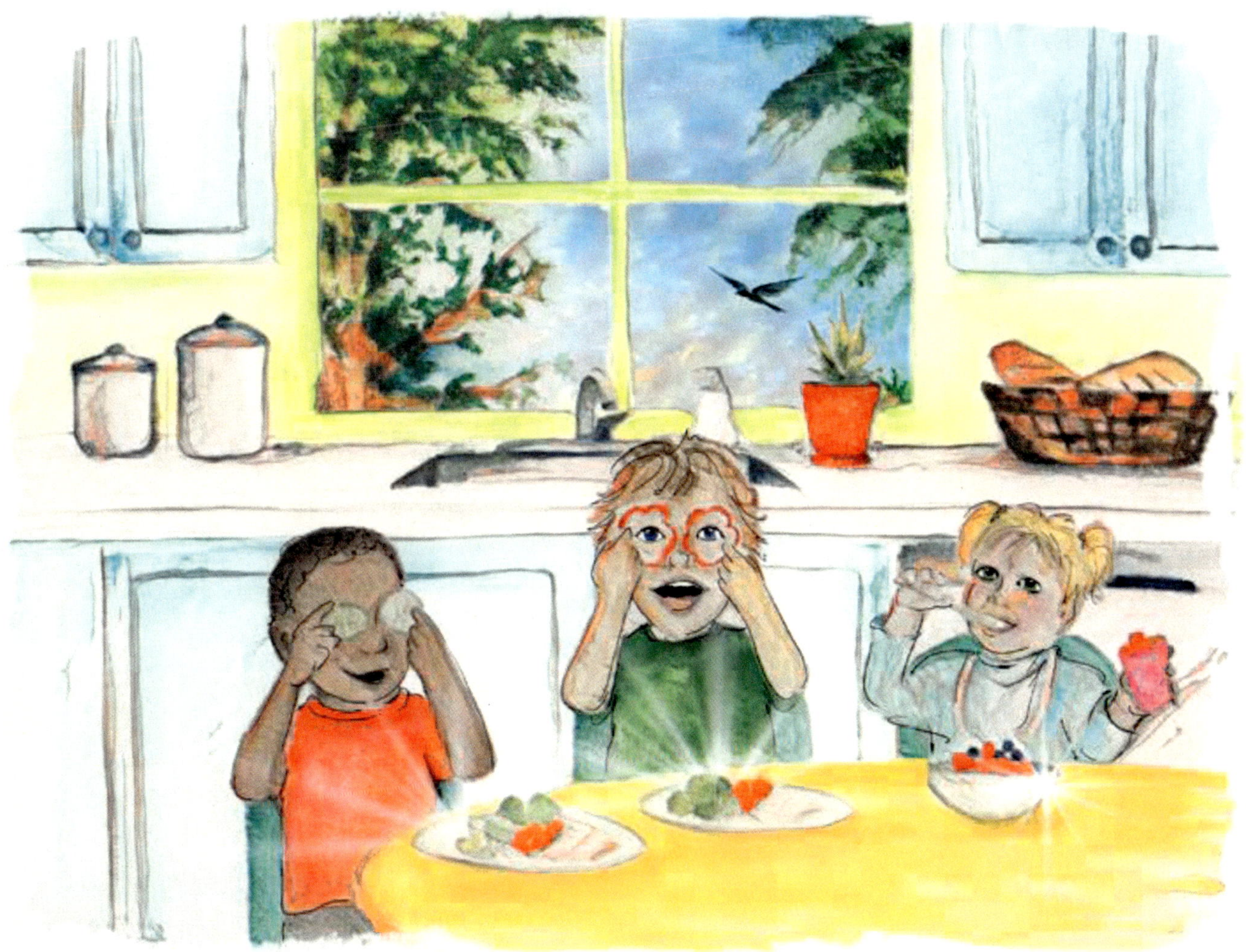

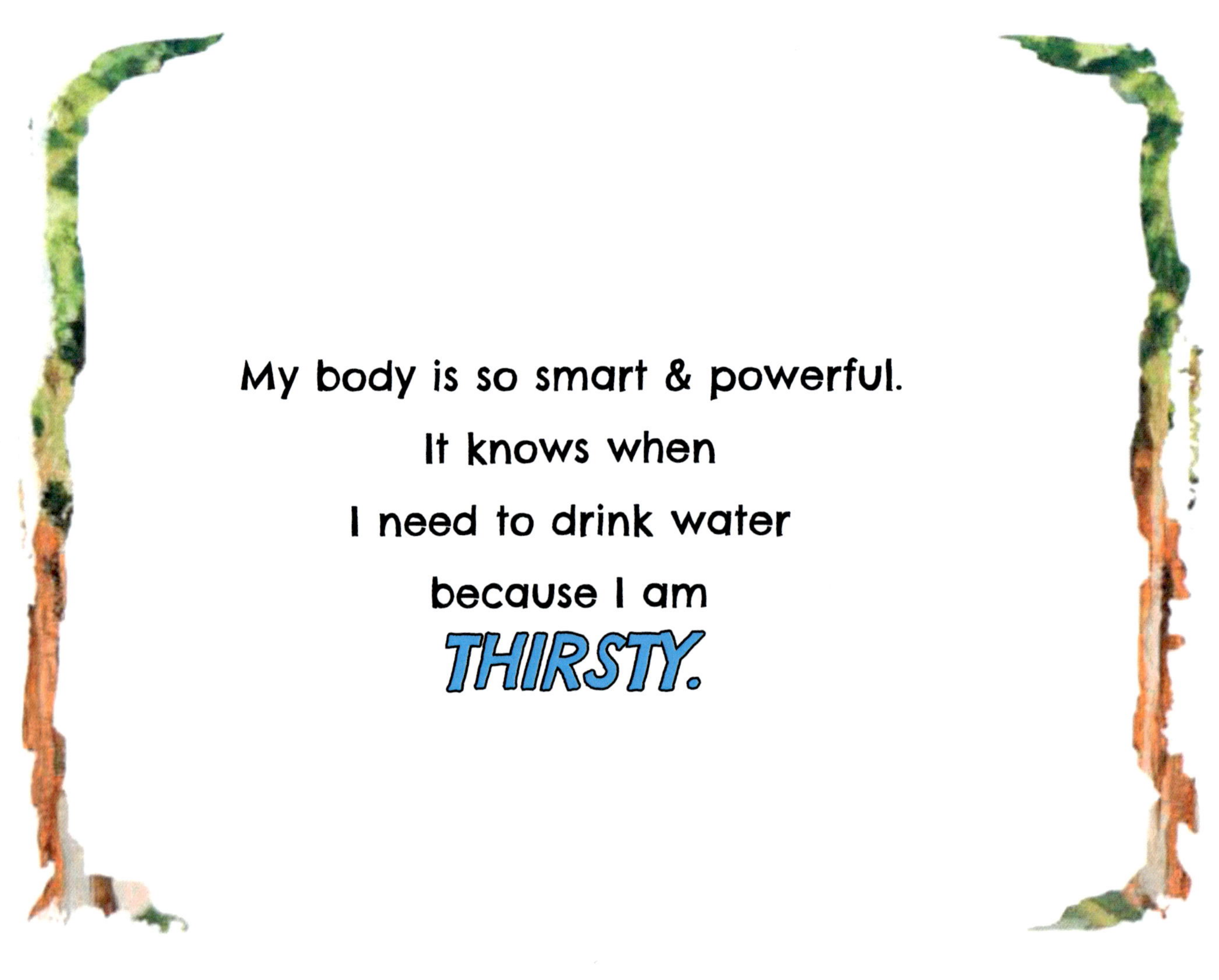

My body is so smart & powerful.

It knows when

I need to drink water

because I am

THIRSTY.

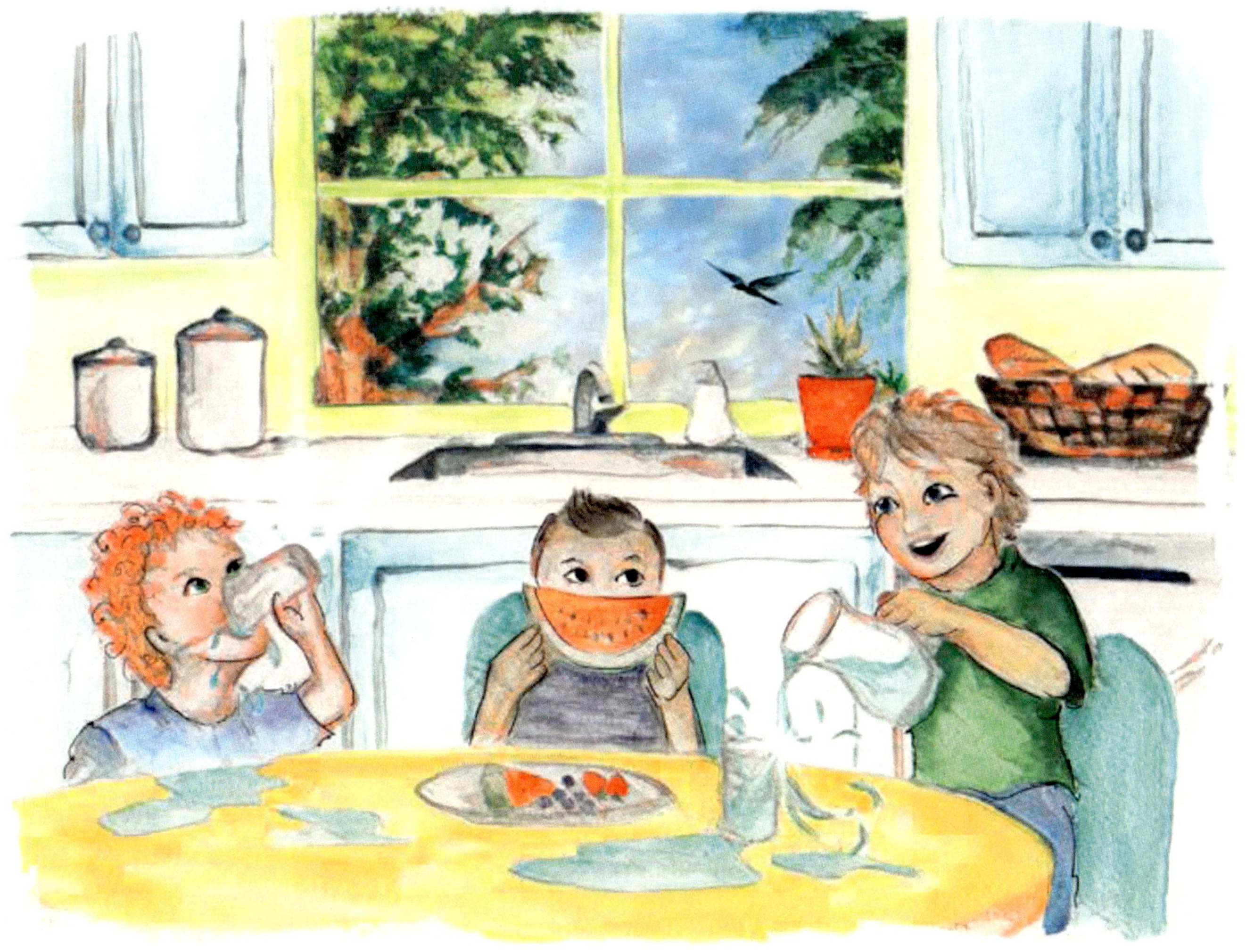

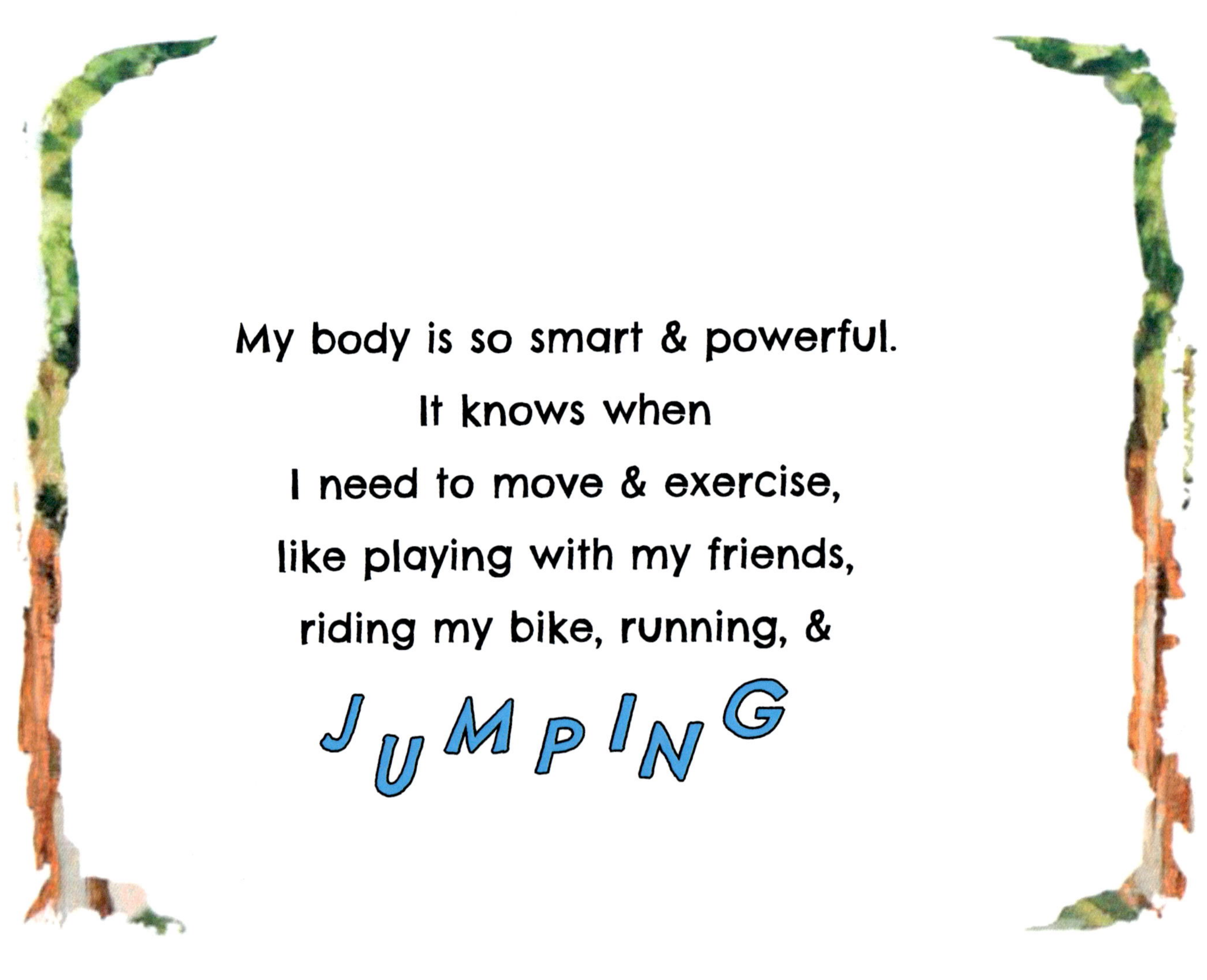

My body is so smart & powerful.

It knows when

I need to move & exercise,

like playing with my friends,

riding my bike, running, &

JUMPING

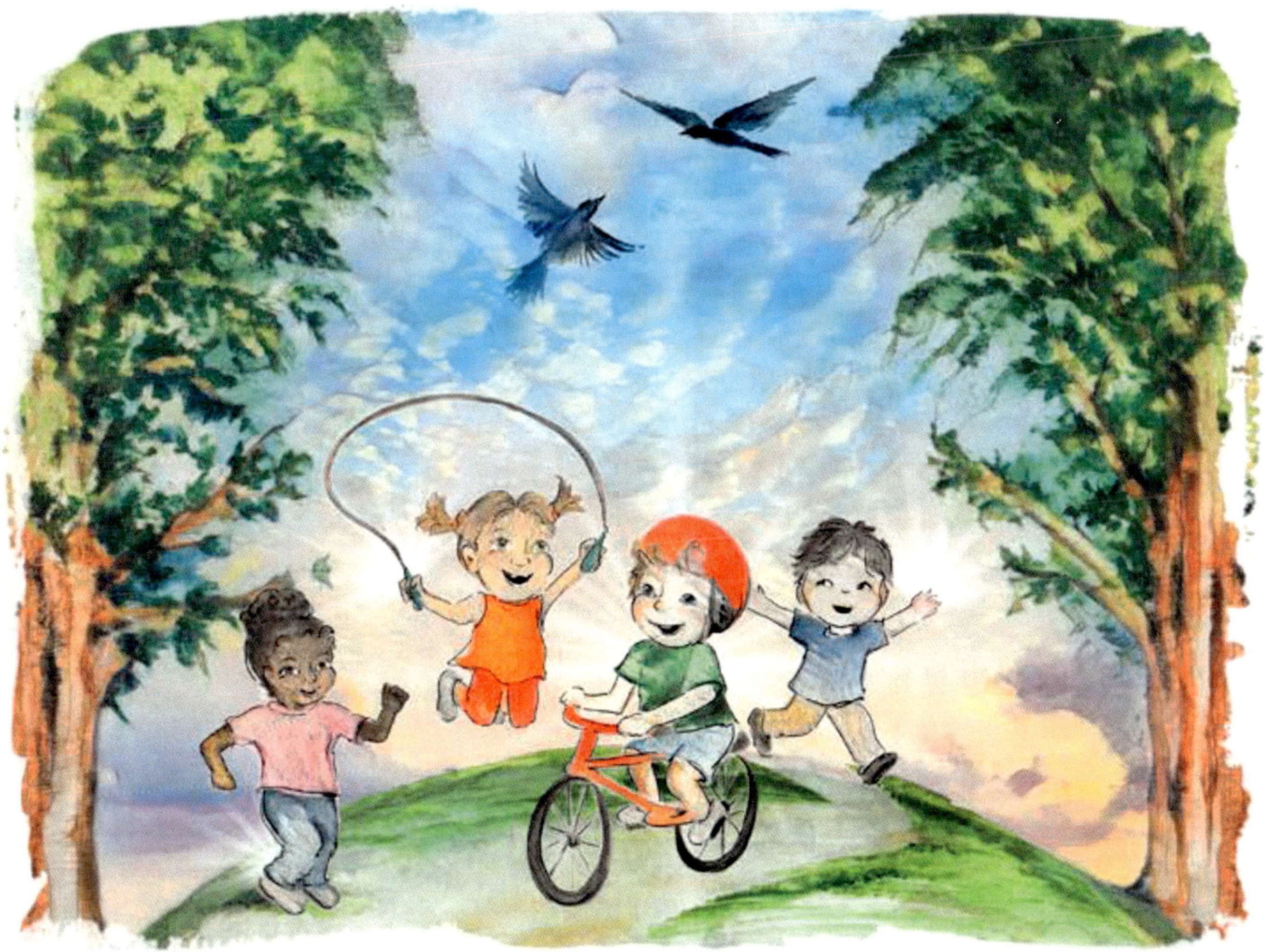

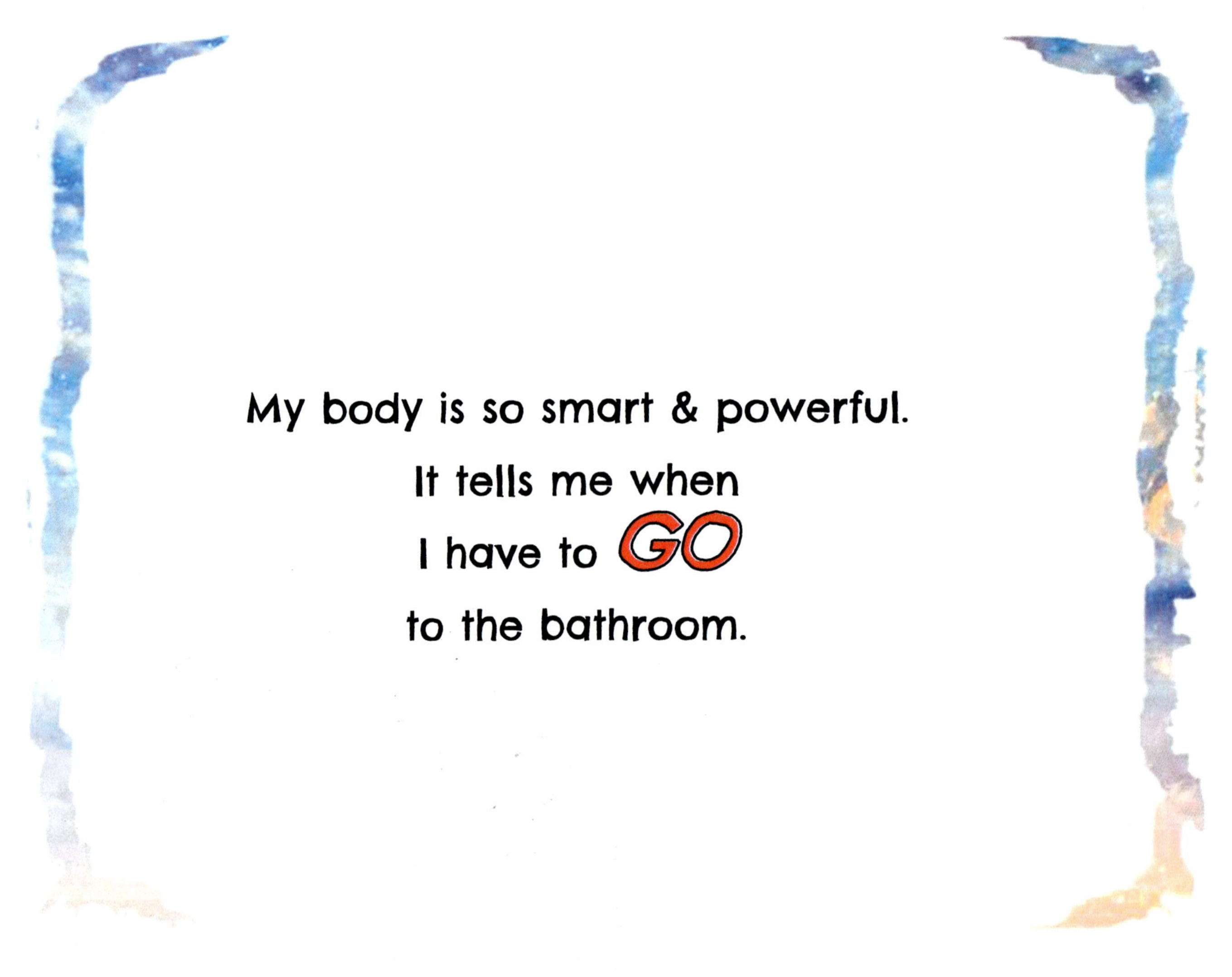

My body is so smart & powerful.

It tells me when

I have to **GO**

to the bathroom.

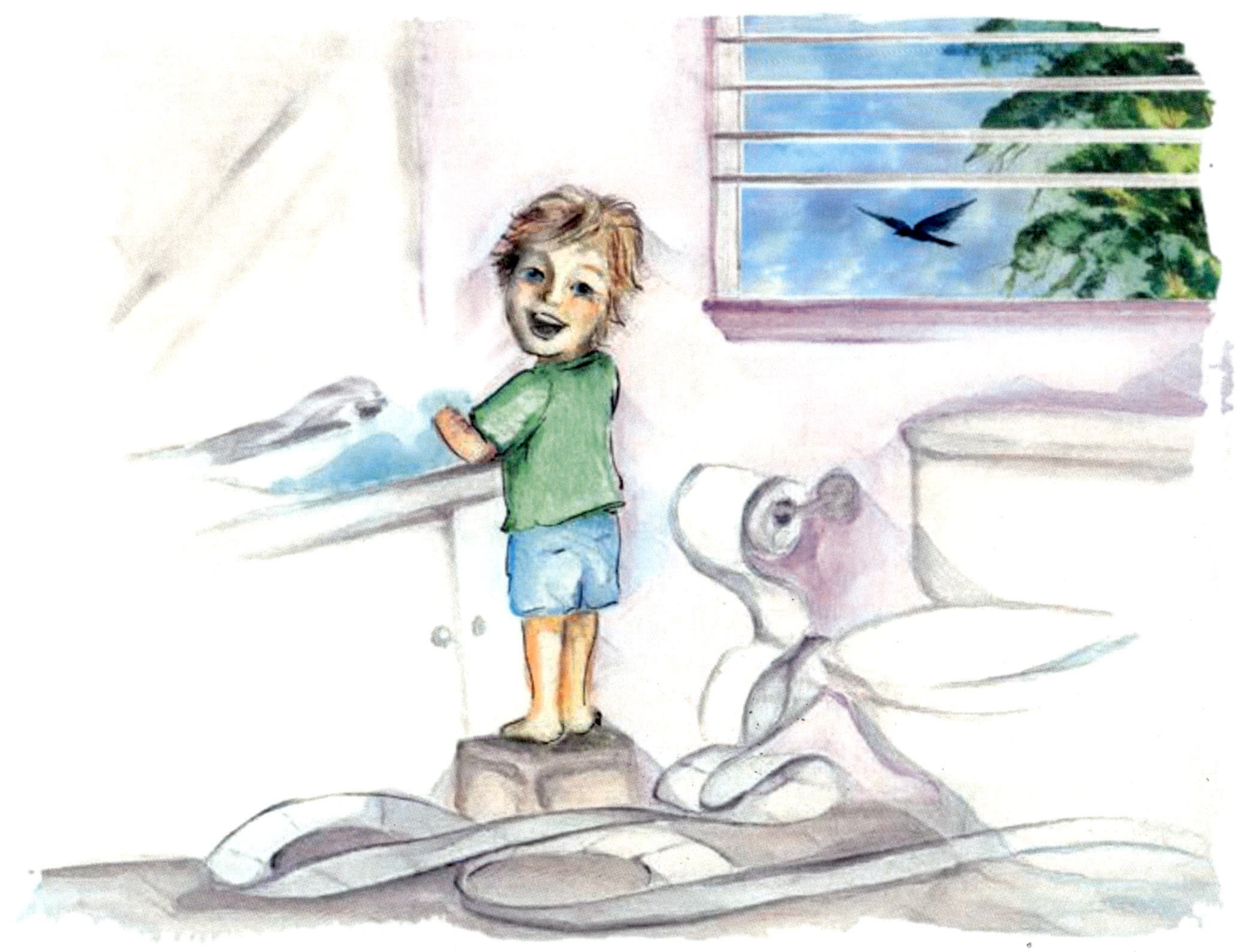

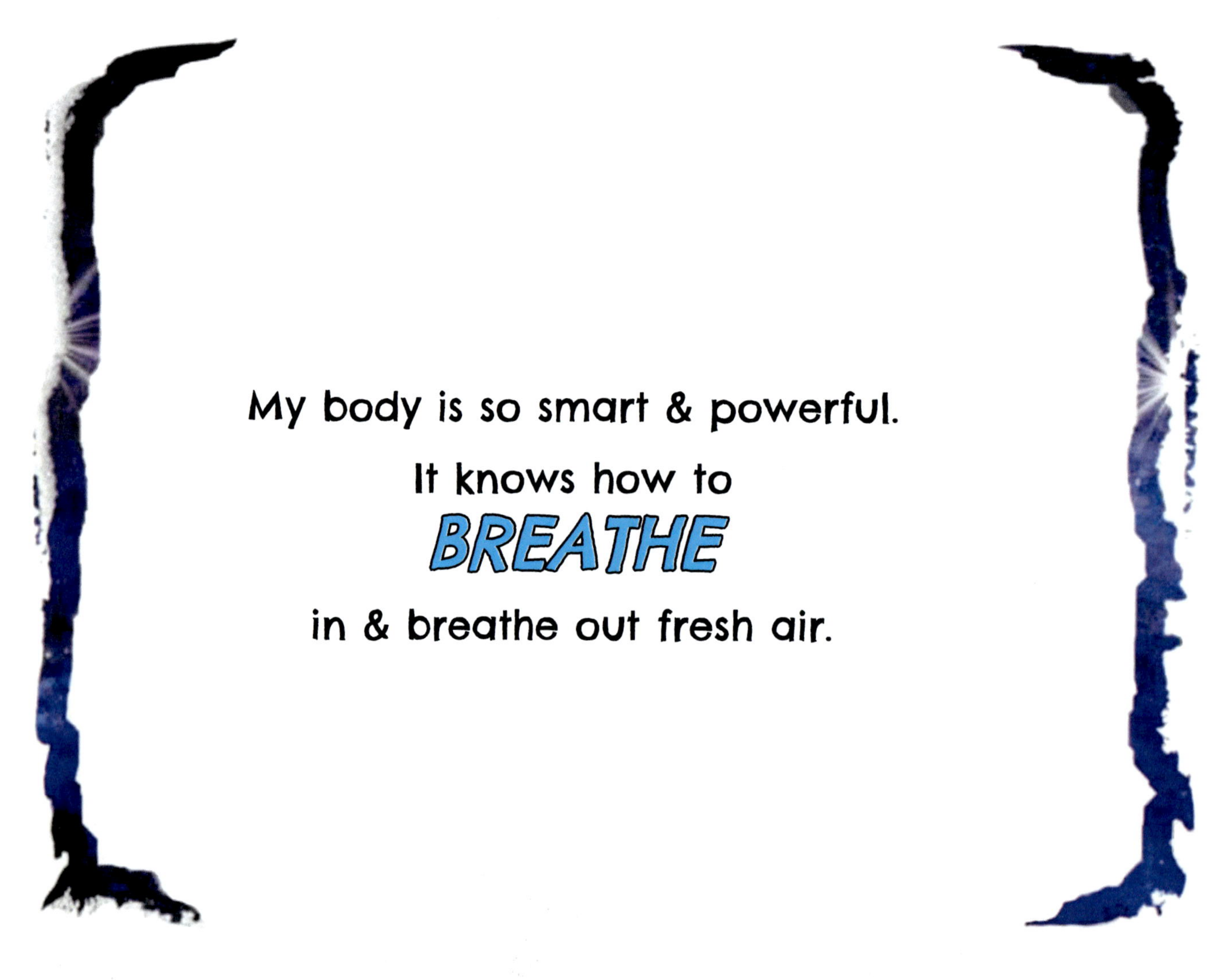

My body is so smart & powerful.

It knows how to

BREATHE

in & breathe out fresh air.

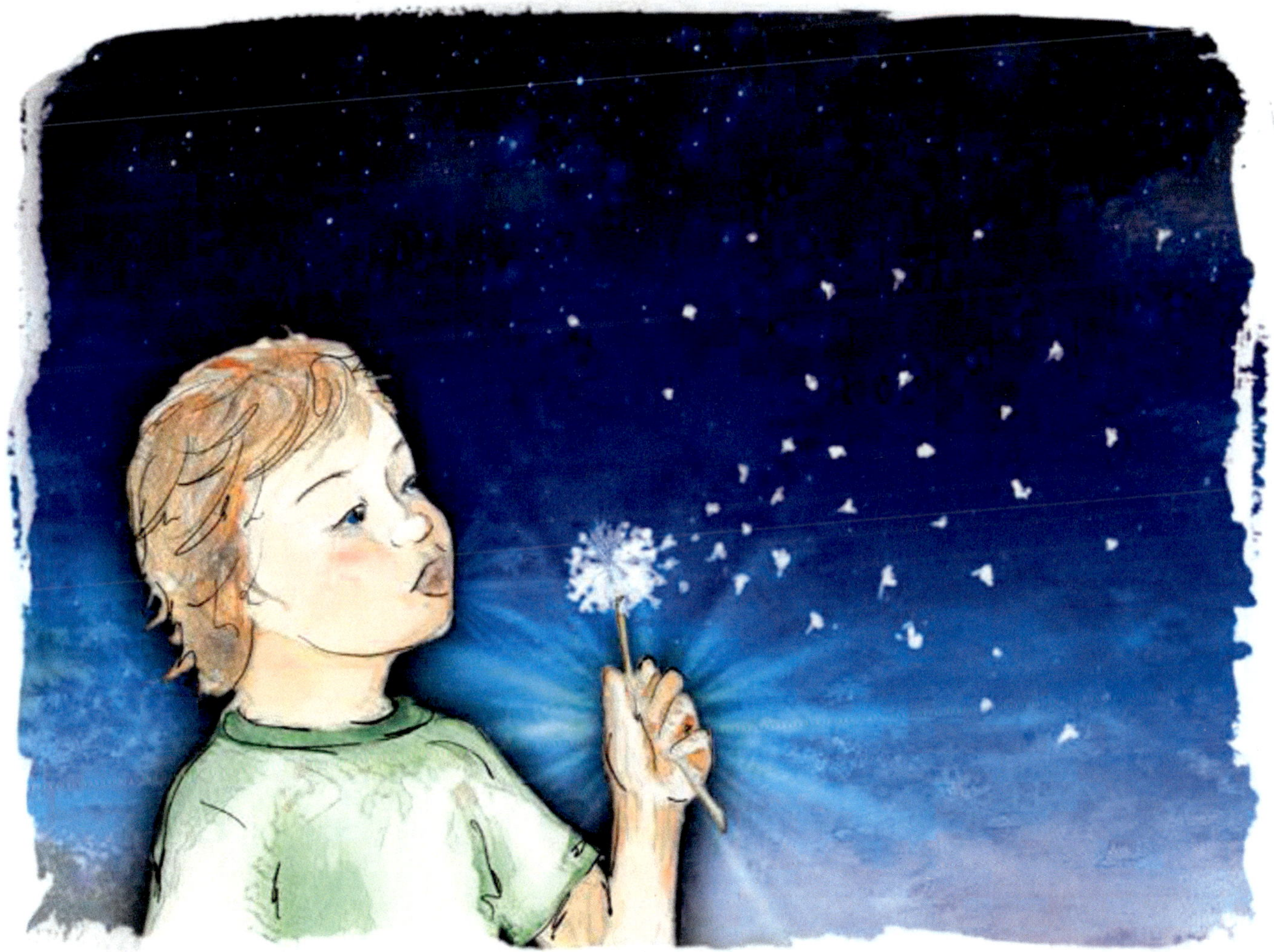

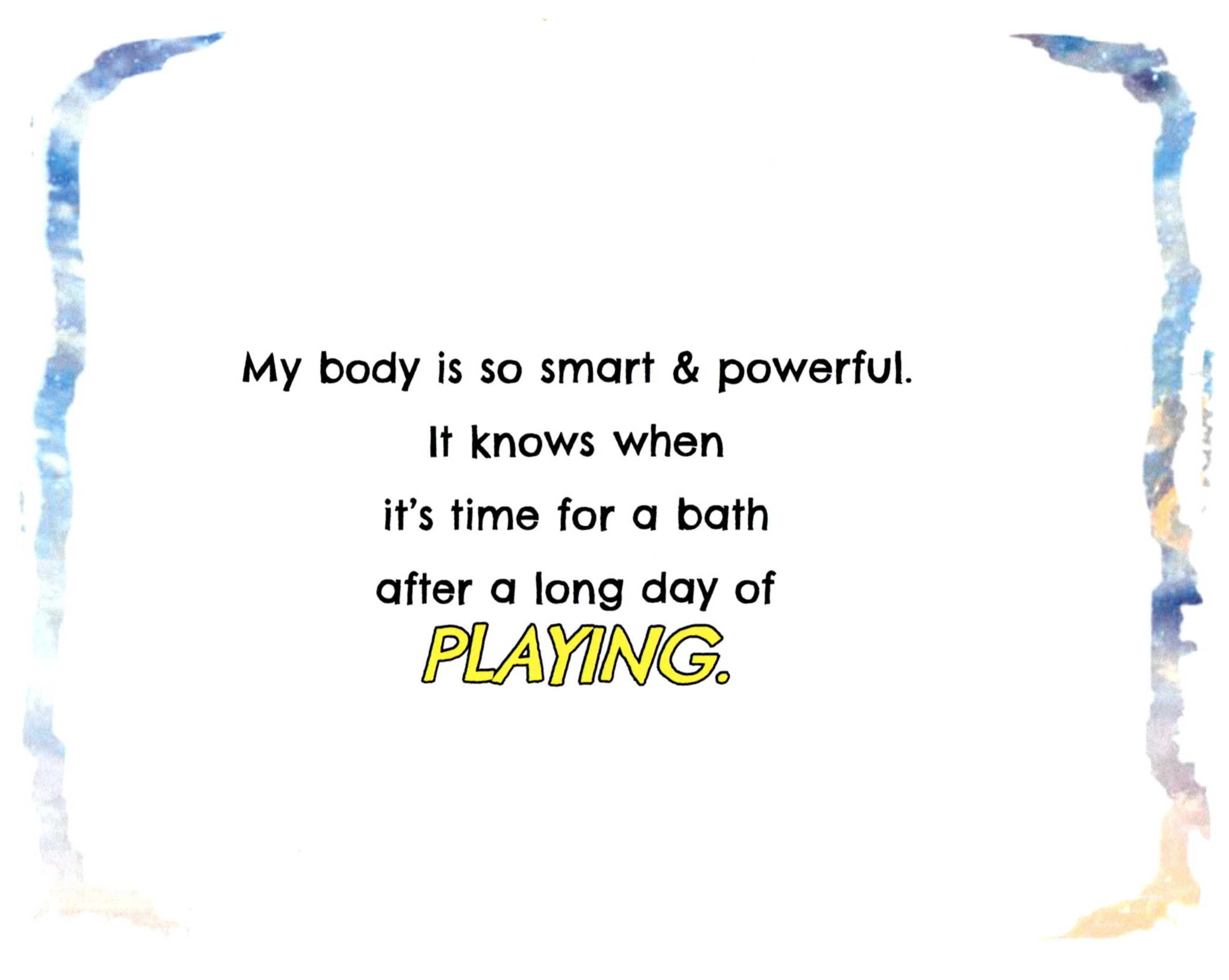

My body is so smart & powerful.
It knows when
it's time for a bath
after a long day of
PLAYING.

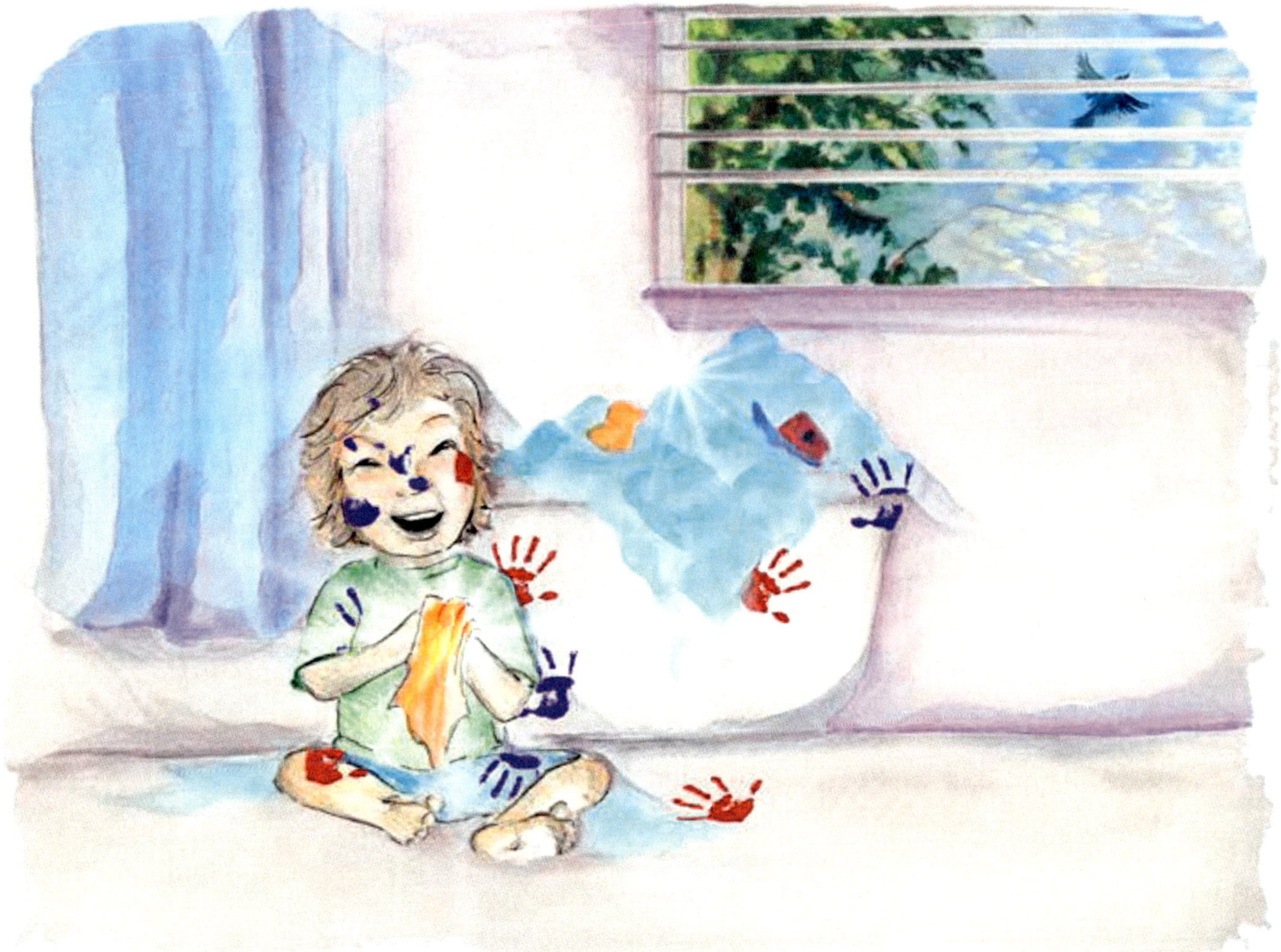

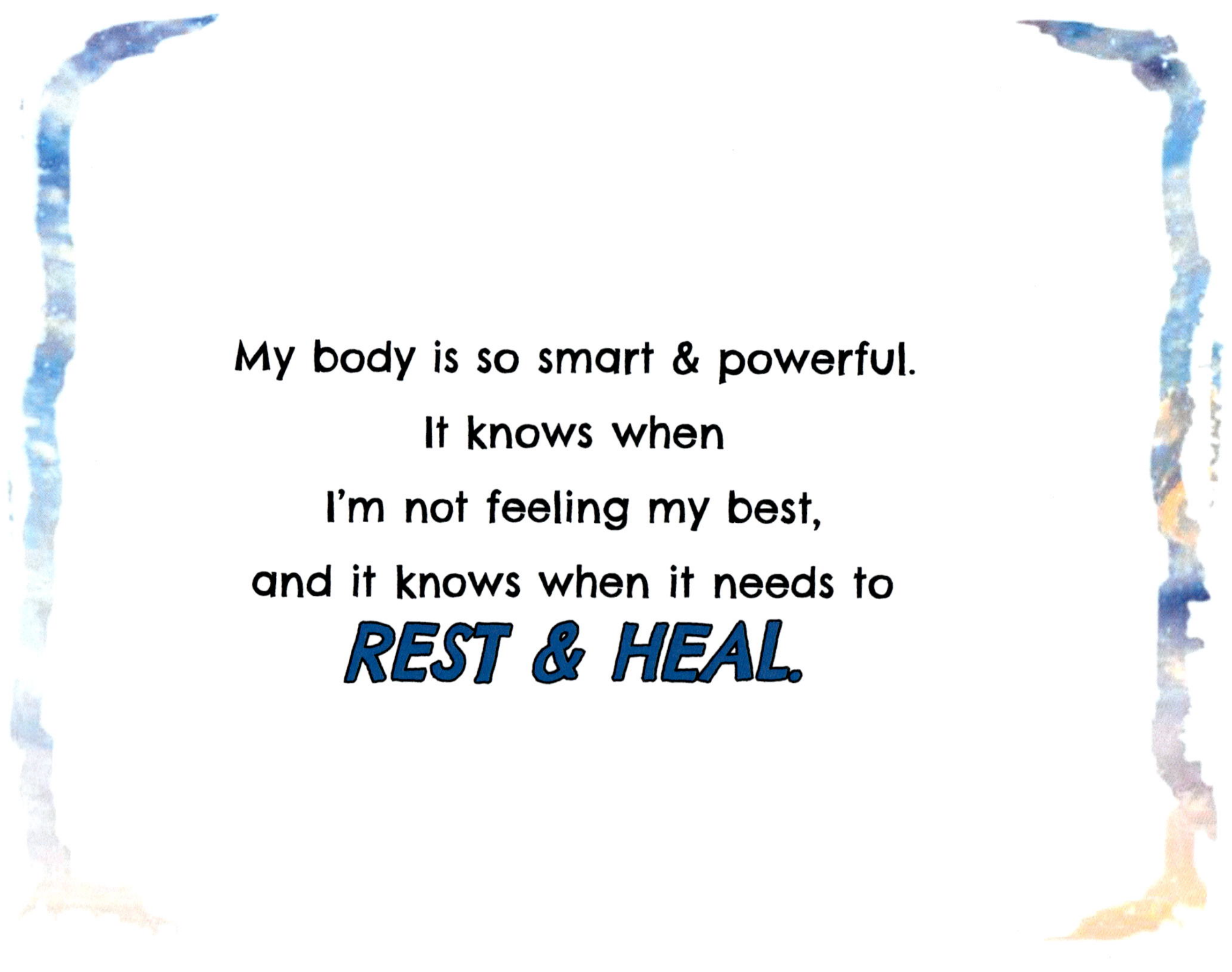

My body is so smart & powerful.
It knows when
I'm not feeling my best,
and it knows when it needs to
REST & HEAL.

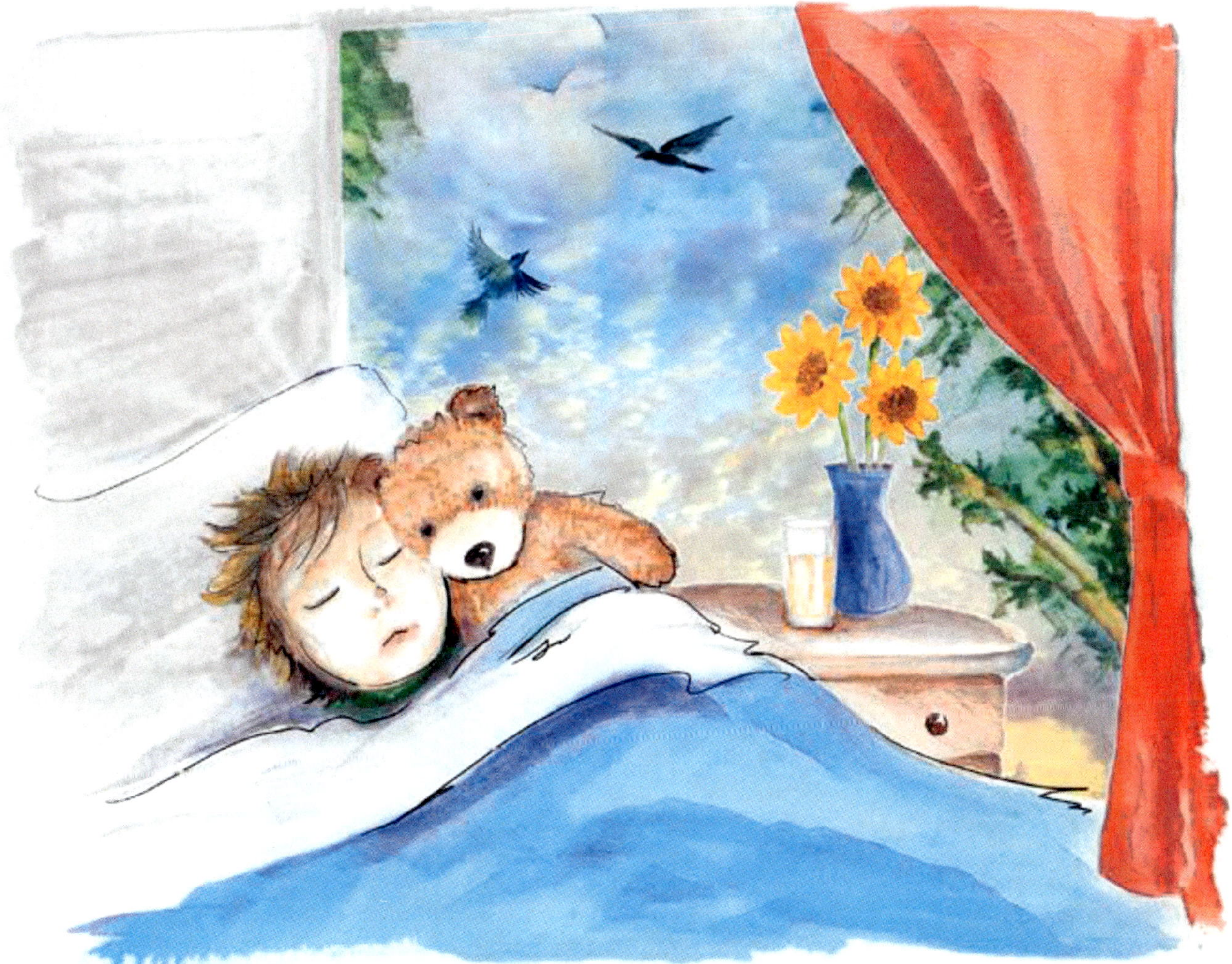

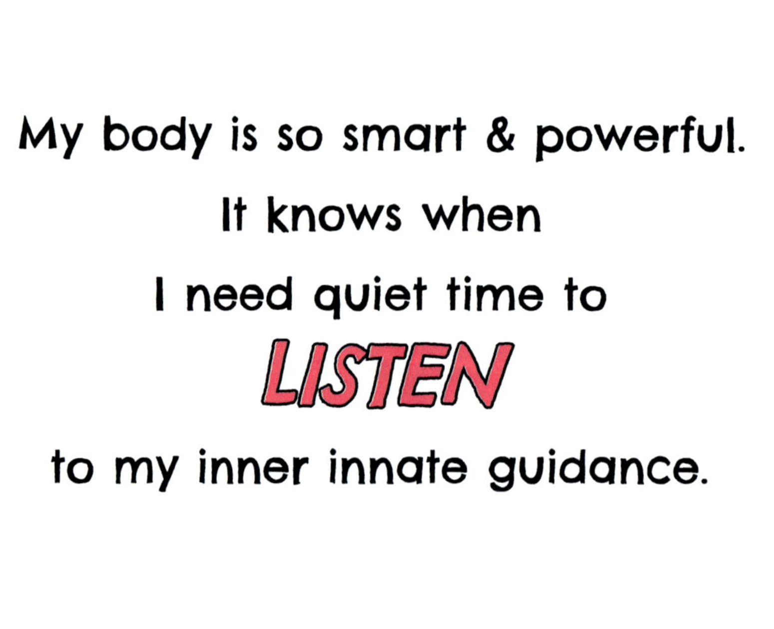

My body is so smart & powerful.

It knows when

I need quiet time to

LISTEN

to my inner innate guidance.

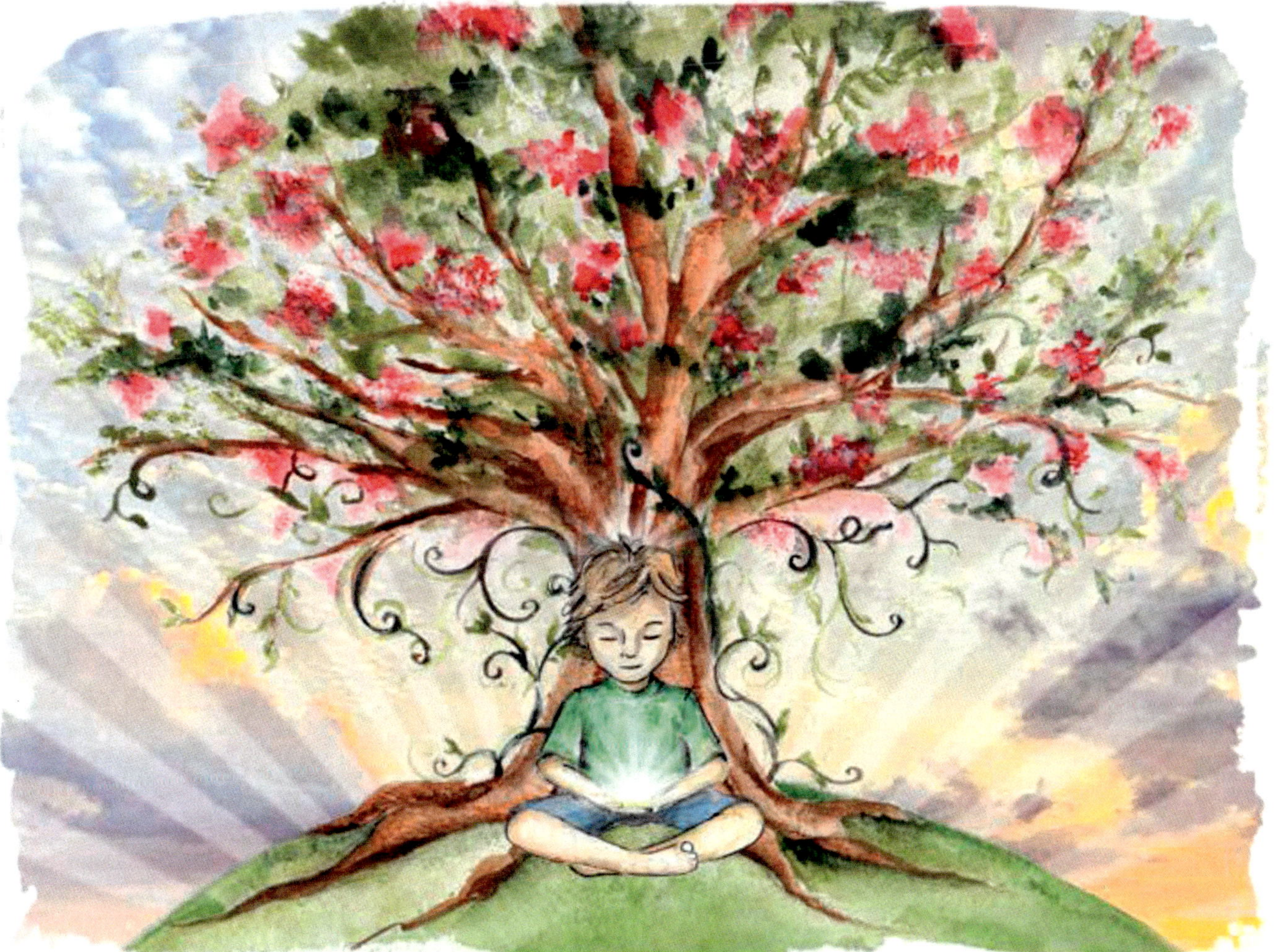

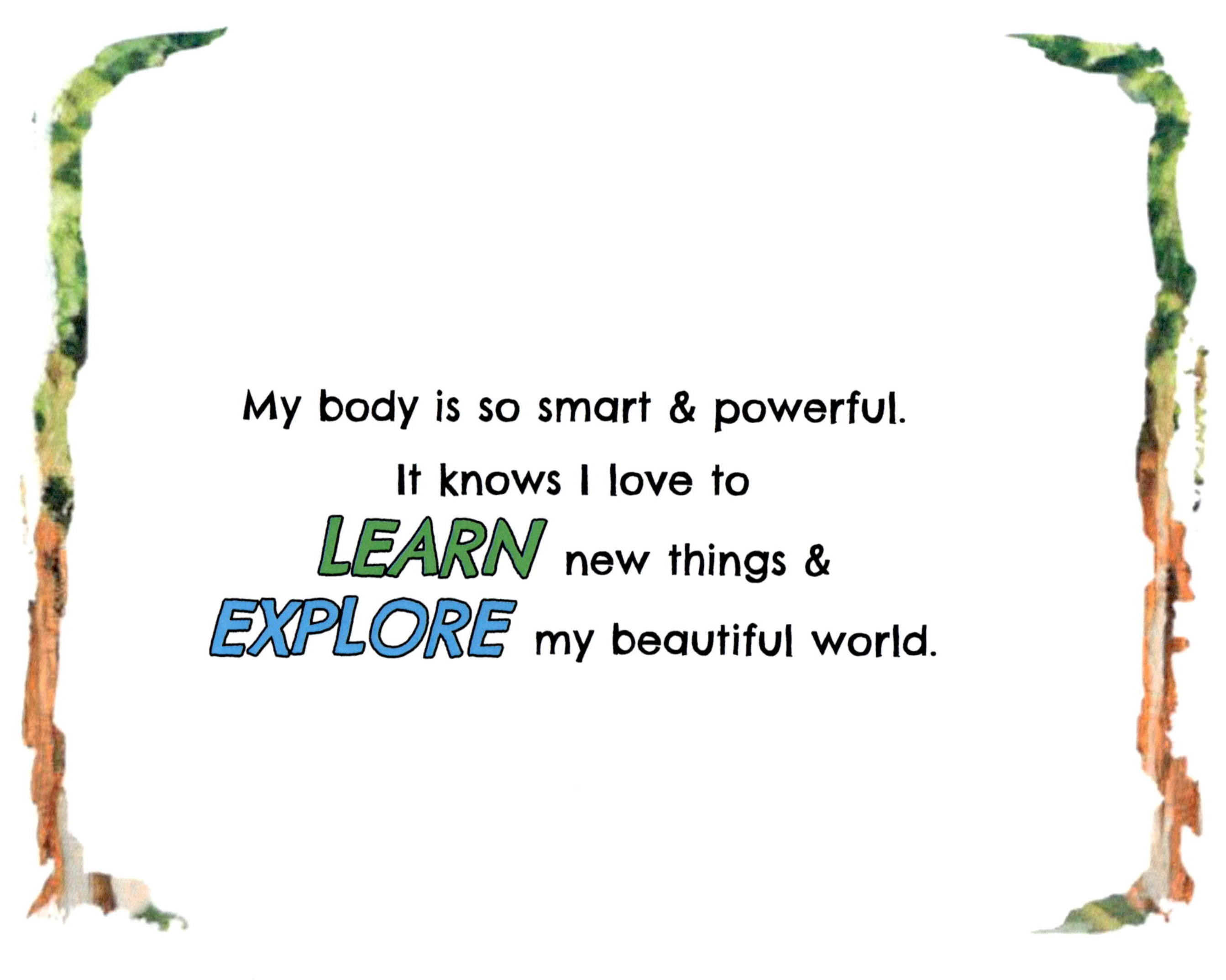

My body is so smart & powerful.

It knows I love to

LEARN new things &

EXPLORE my beautiful world.

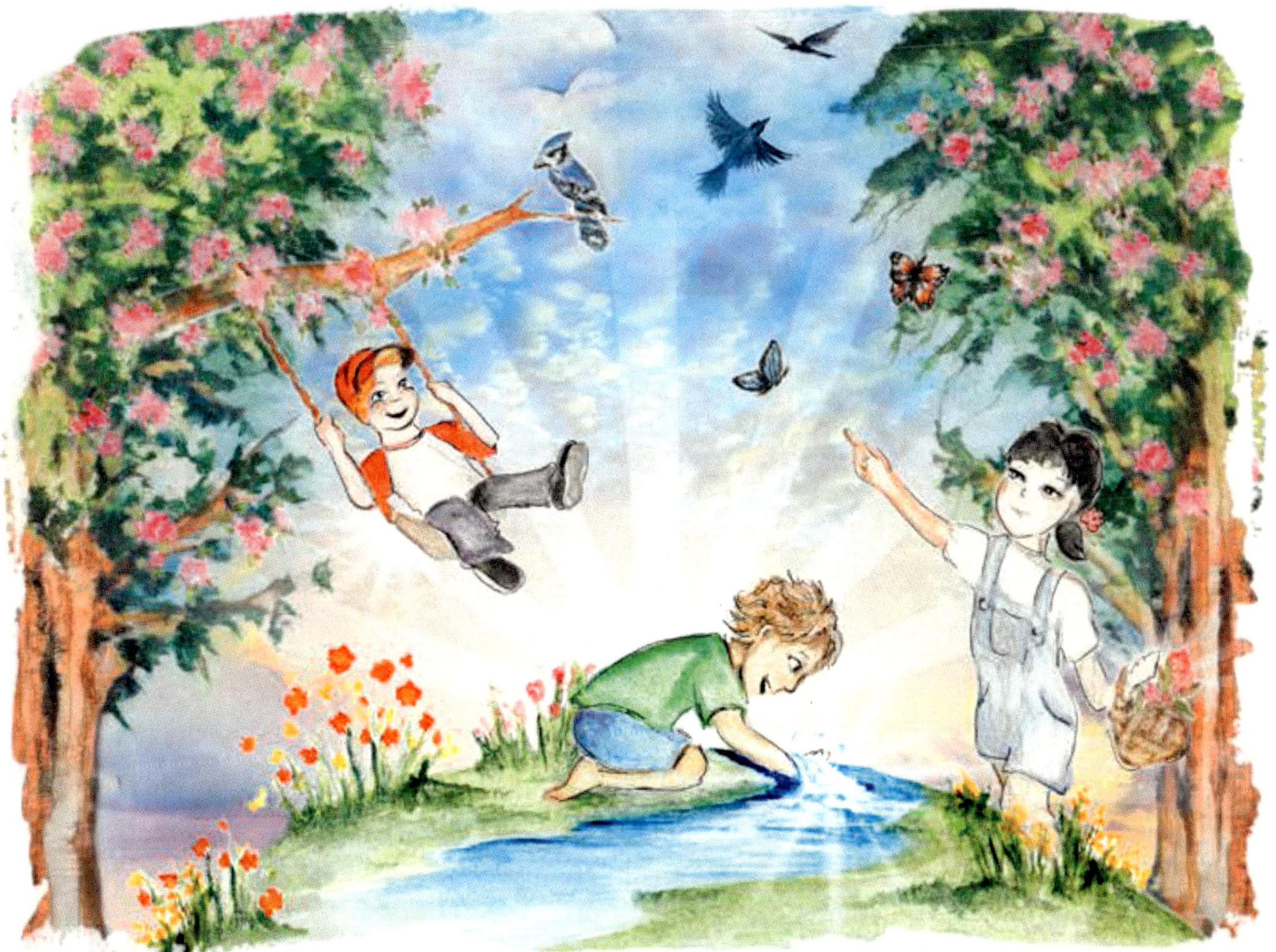

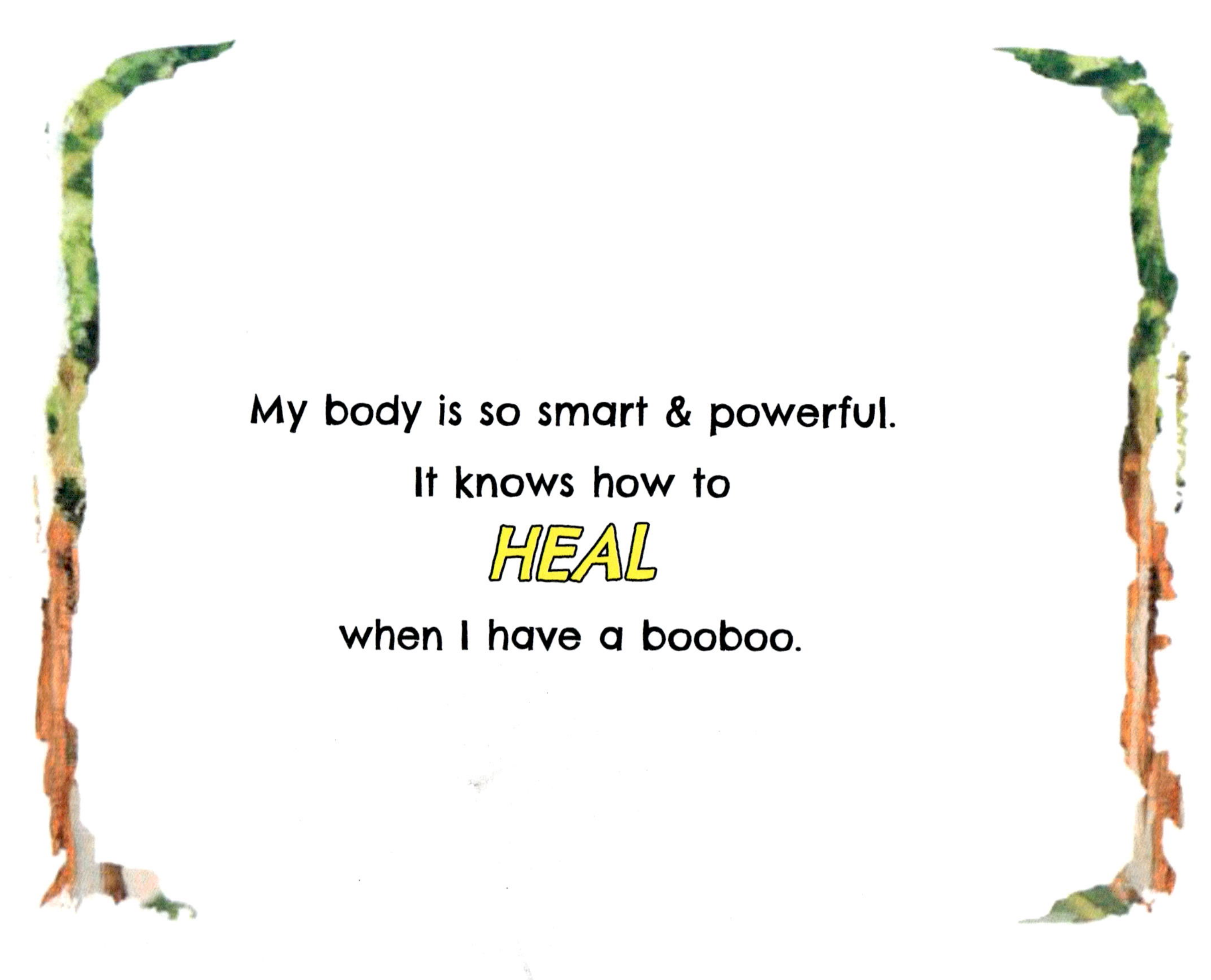

My body is so smart & powerful.

It knows how to

HEAL

when I have a booboo.

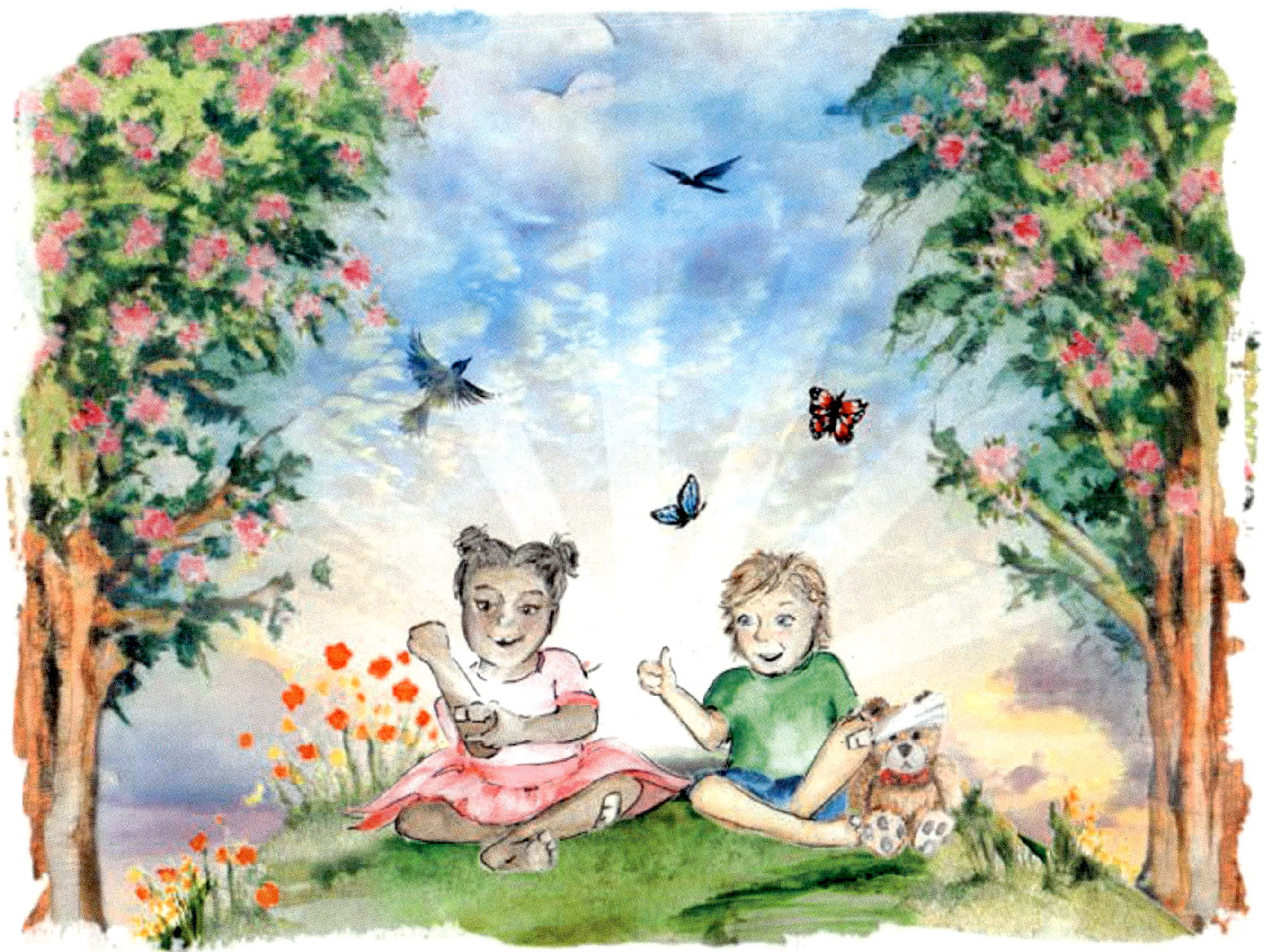

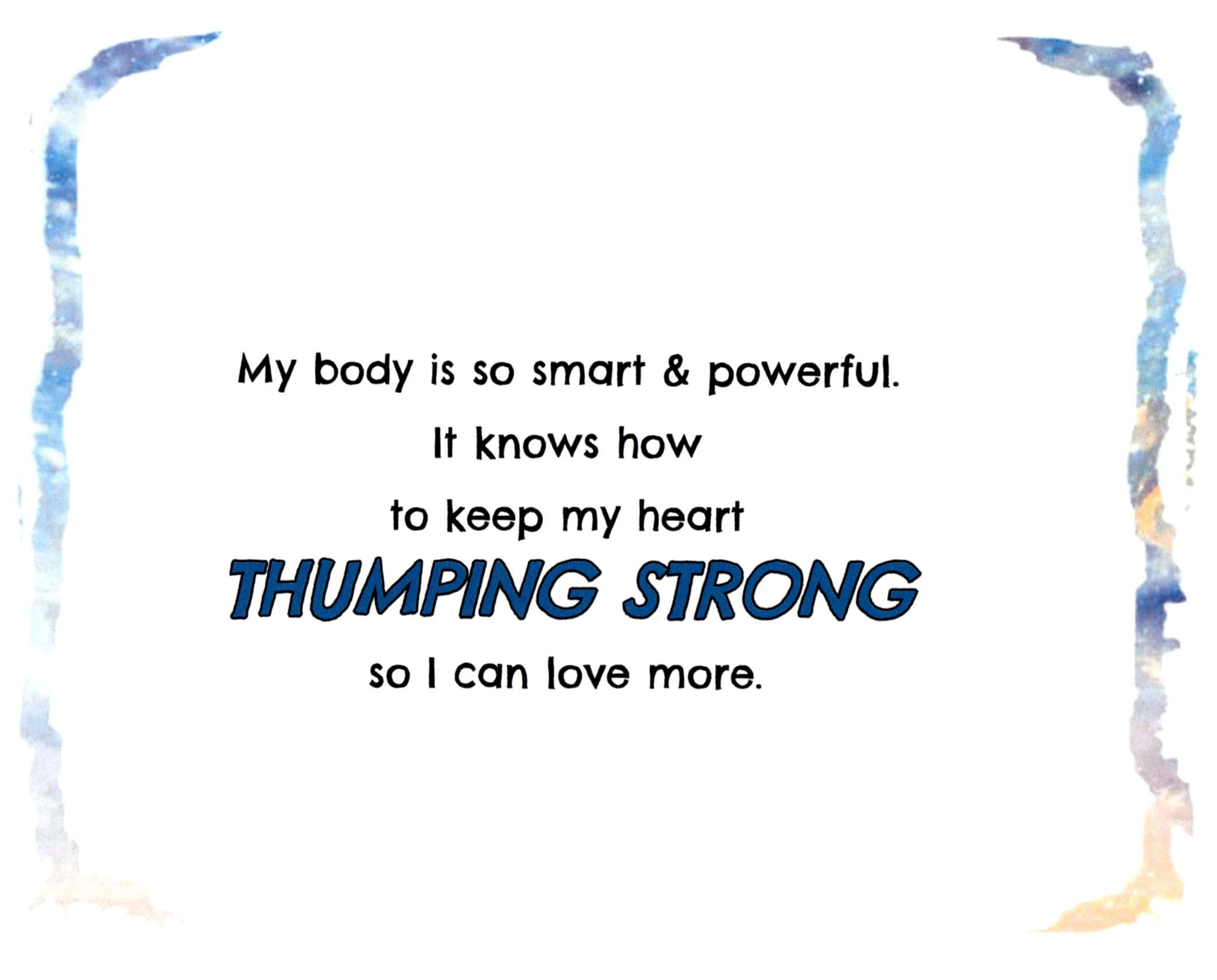

My body is so smart & powerful.
It knows how
to keep my heart
THUMPING STRONG
so I can love more.

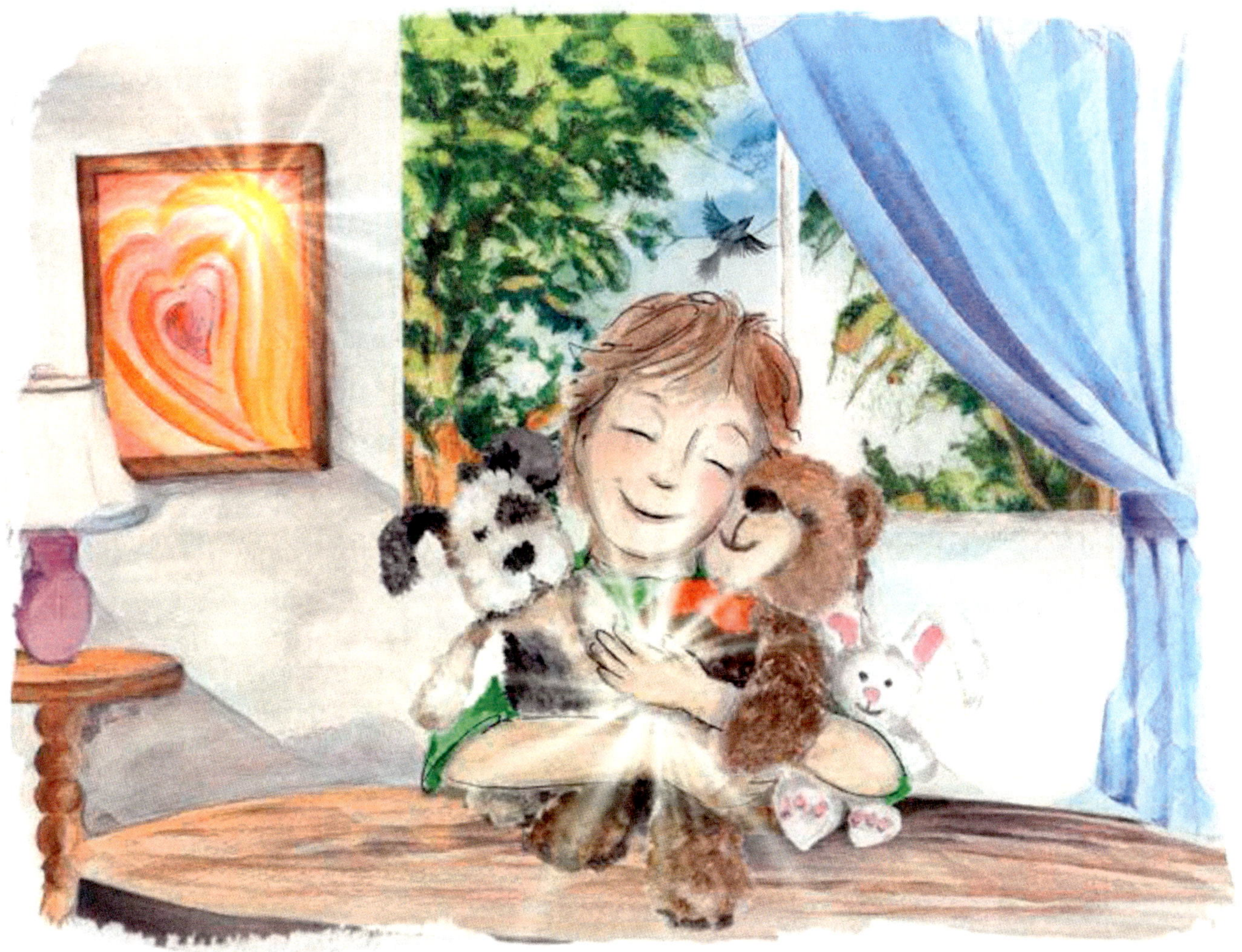

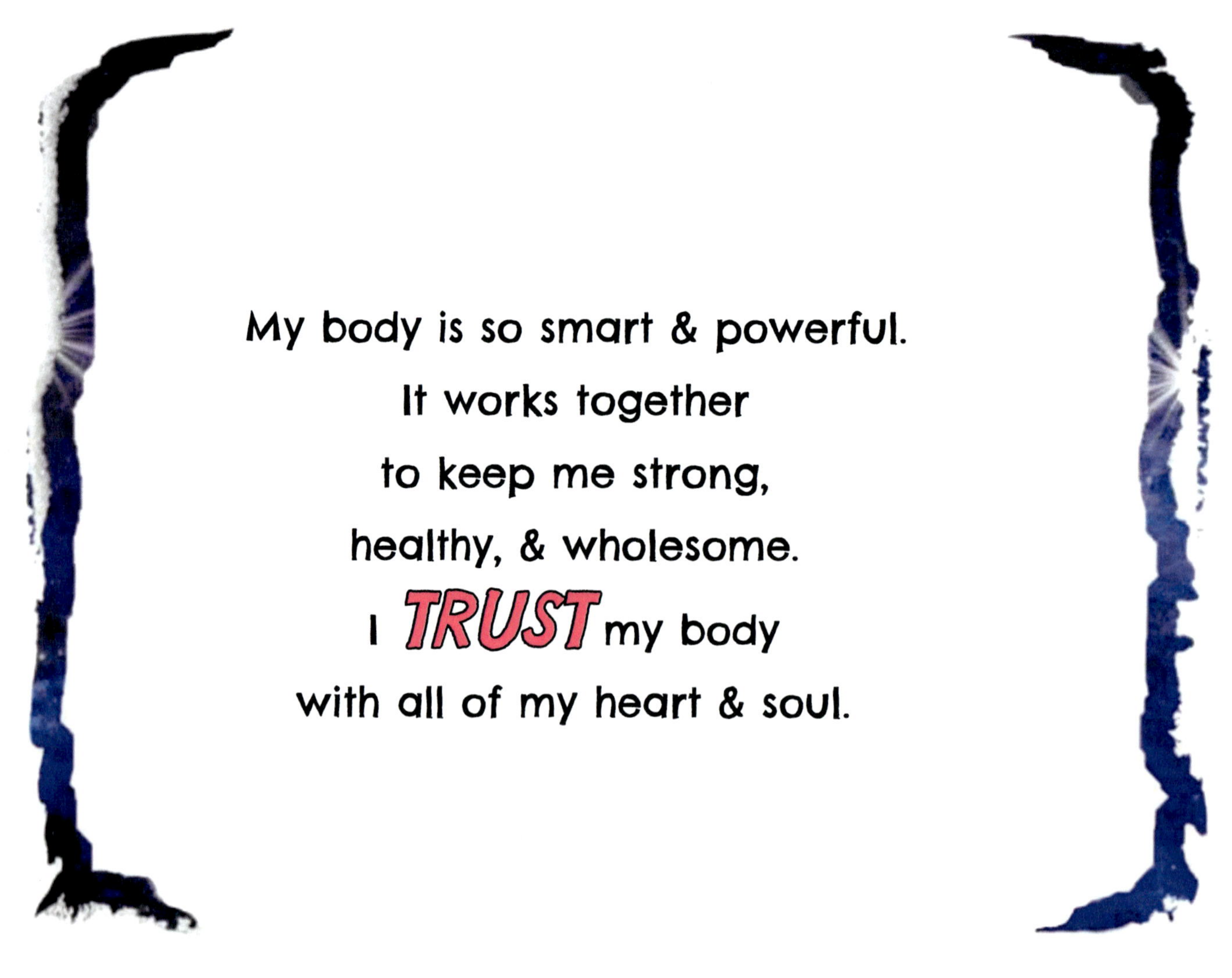

My body is so smart & powerful.
It works together
to keep me strong,
healthy, & wholesome.
I TRUST my body
with all of my heart & soul.

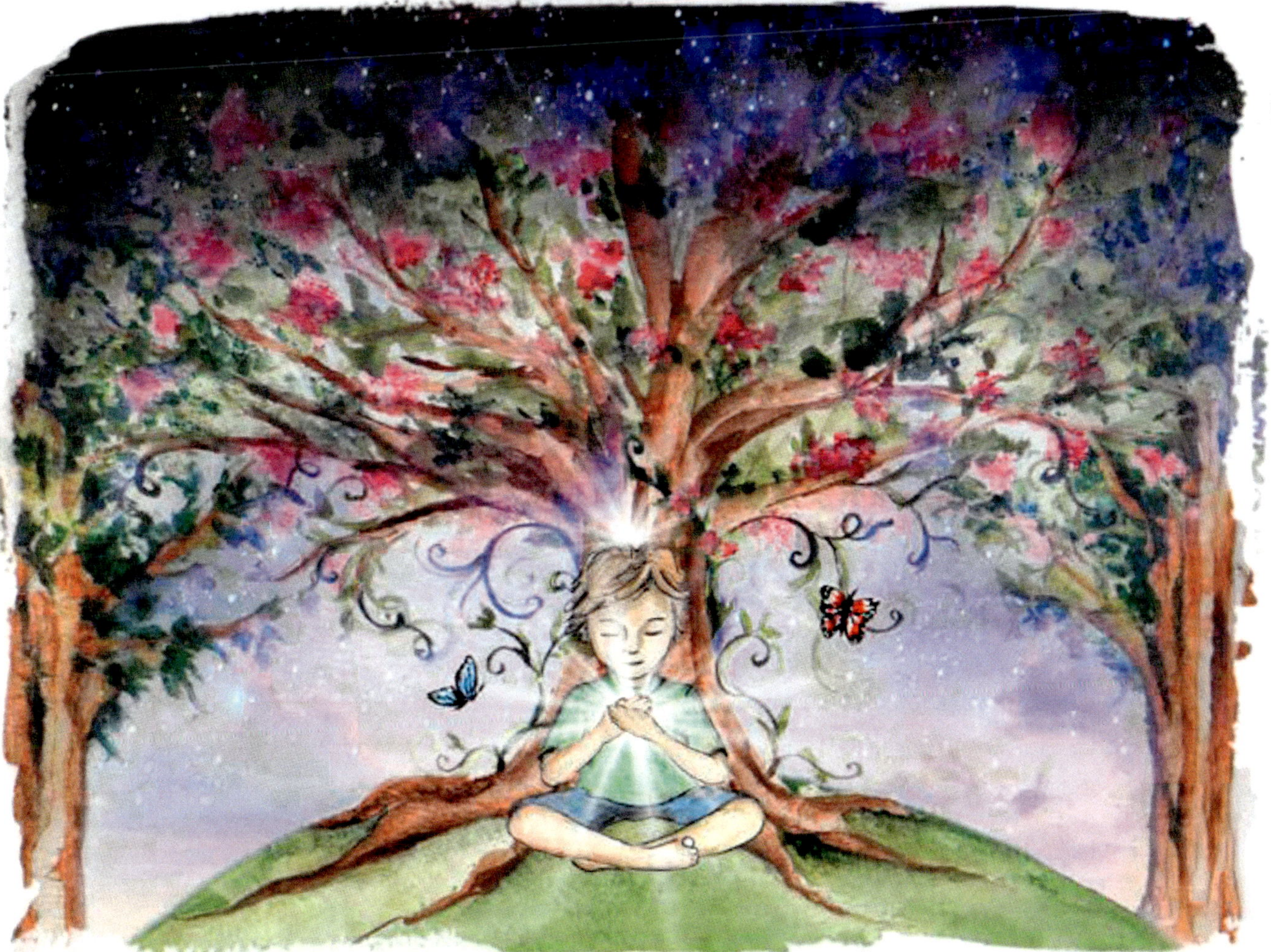

AUTHOR

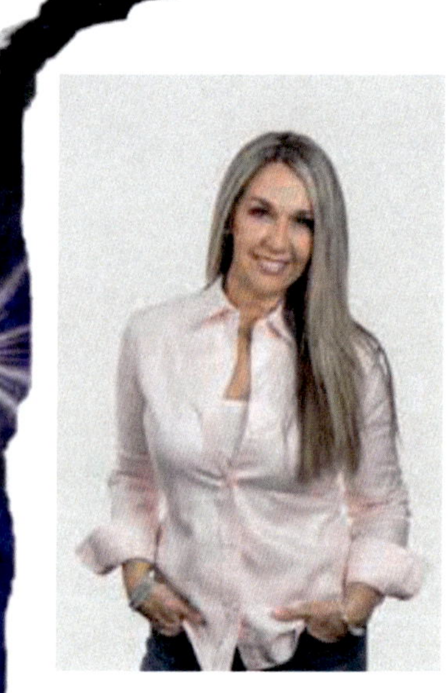

Dr. Patty Cosmelli is a 1993 graduate of Life University and has been in private practice in Tampa, FL, since 1995. She is not only committed to chiropractic but also to a holistic perspective when it comes to optimum health. Dr. Cosmelli's approach to health includes the synergistic relationship between body, mind, and lifestyle.

Dr. Cosmelli focuses on the care of children, including special needs children, as well as expecting moms. She has extensive training in the understanding and care of pediatric patients, with results that are notable and positive. Dr. Cosmelli has published several articles featured in the Chiropractic Journal, which highlight her passion for creating leadership amongst women in the chiropractic profession. She is currently working on her first book and anticipates publishing and release at a later date. Dr. Cosmelli is frequently sought after as a speaker and has spoken at several chiropractic venues as an inspirational lecturer, especially to women who need guidance and reassurance. Her leadership has been noted not only professionally but also on a personal level.

Dr. Patty Cosmelli's professional affiliations include the following:

Co-Founder of an all-women's chiropractic organization

Past Co-President of The League of Chiropractic Women

ILLUSTRATOR

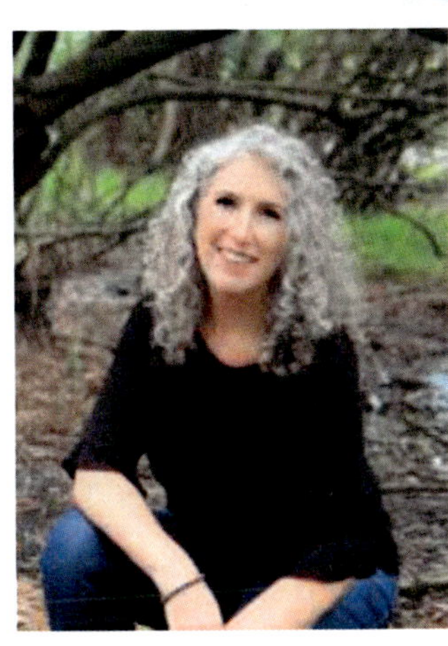

Christina M. Kusek is a multifaceted artist known for her vibrant use of color, captivating detail and ability to illuminate an image that speaks to the heart. Originally from New Jersey, she has lived in Florida since 2008, where she works as Senior Manager, CAD to create one-of-a-kind wearable art for a global women's fashion brand. She holds a BFA with honors from the College of Visual and Performing Arts, School of Art and Design at Syracuse University, and began her career as a surface pattern designer for home fashions in New York City. Christina is driven by a deep passion for helping children and adults through her artwork. For more than 20 years she has enjoyed honing her craft as an energy artist and illustrator. Dubbed "the Dreamer" by her friends and family, Christina is committed to helping people find their true heart's center.

Write What You Like About YOU!

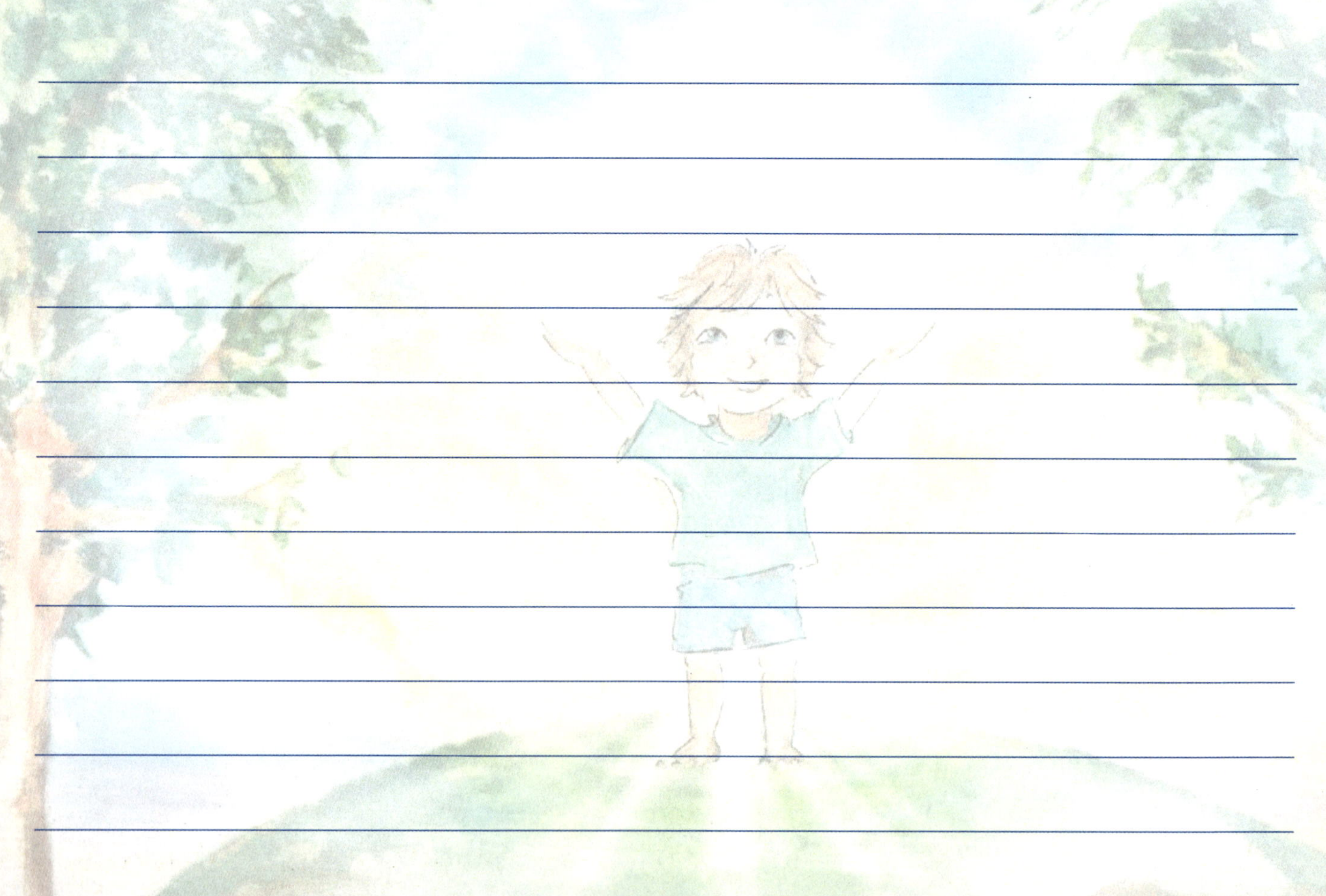

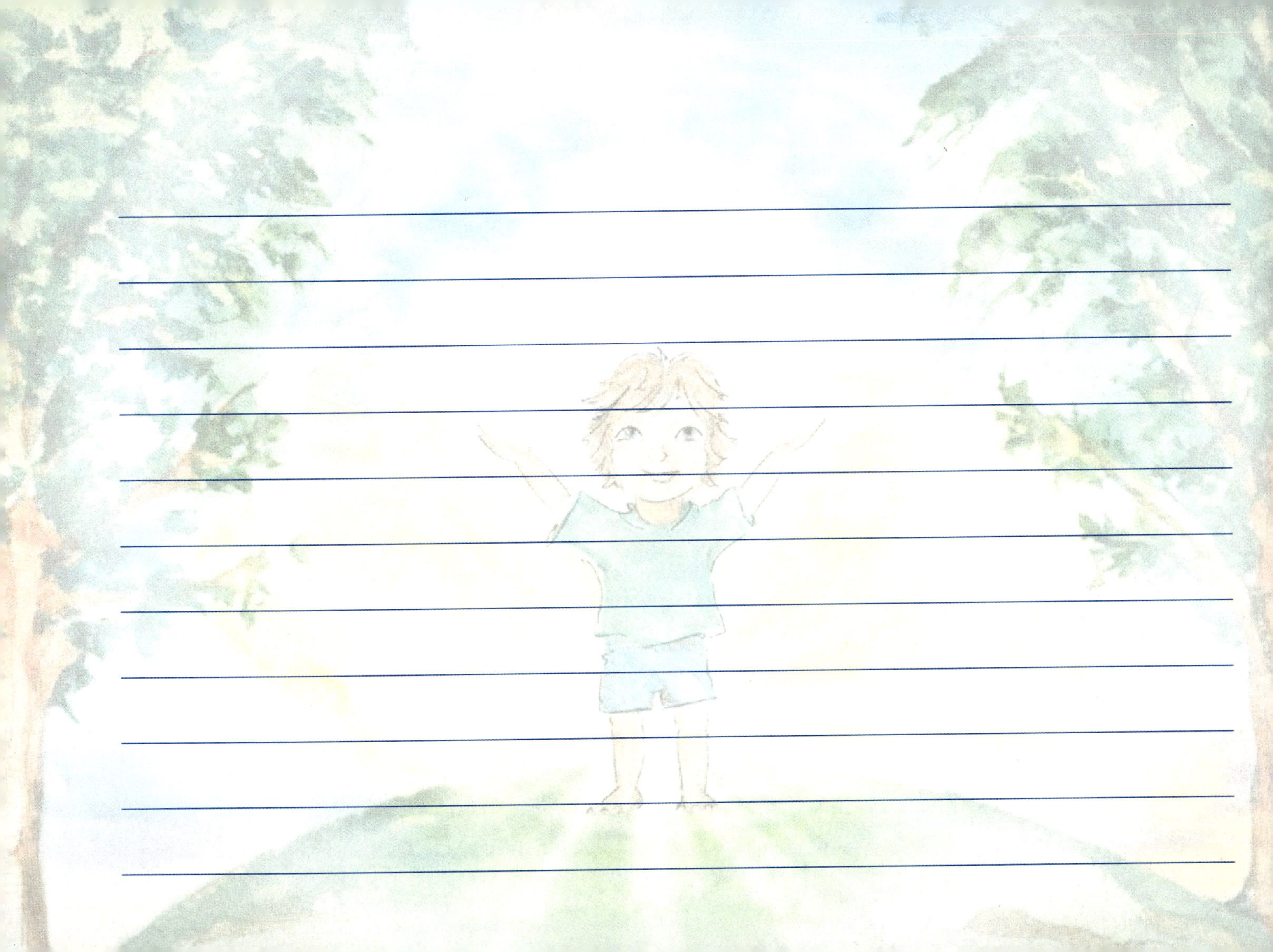

Made in United States
Orlando, FL
26 August 2023